Illustratec
for Mig1
Acupuncture, M
and Tuina Massage

of related interest

Illustrated Treatment for Cervical Spondylosis Using Massage Therapy
Tang Xuezhang and Yu Tianyuan
ISBN 978 1 84819 062 7

Tuina/ Massage Manipulations
Basic Principles and Techniques
Chief Editor: Li Jiangshan
ISBN 978 1 84819 058 0

Needling Techniques for Acupuncturists
Basic Principles and Techniques
Chief Editor: Professor Chang Xiaorong
ISBN 978 1 84819 057 3

Basic Theories of Traditional Chinese Medicine
Edited by Zhu Bing and Wang Hongcai
Advisor: Cheng Xinnong
ISBN 978 1 84819 038 2

Diagnostics of Traditional Chinese Medicine
Edited by Zhu Bing and Wang Hongcai
Advisor: Cheng Xinnong
ISBN 978 1 84819 036 8

Meridians and Acupoints
Edited by Zhu Bing and Wang Hongcai
Advisor: Cheng Xinnong
ISBN 978 1 84819 037 5

Acupuncture Therapeutics
Edited by Zhu Bing and Wang Hongcai
Advisor: Cheng Xinnong
ISBN 978 1 84819 039 9

Case Studies from the Medical Records of Leading
Chinese Acupuncture Experts
Edited by Zhu Bing and Wang Hongcai
Advisor: Cheng Xinnong
ISBN 978 1 84819 046 7

Illustrated Treatment for Migraine Using Acupuncture, Moxibustion and Tuina Massage

Cui Chengbin and Xing Xiaomin

SINGING DRAGON

LONDON AND PHILADELPHIA

Associate Editors: Meng Fanguang, Li Xiubin and Ma Liangzhi
Committee Members: Cui Chengbin, Xing Xiaomin, Meng Fanguang, Li Xiubin, Ma Liangzhi, Jiao Yue, Hu Jing, Li Jian, Ji Pingping, Zhou Yong, Li Xudong, Zou Nan, Qin Wenying, Shi Yuhong, Cheng Yunxia, Han Dongmei and Astrid Schmidt
English Supervisor: Michele Ball
Translators: Jing Meng, Wang Jing and Wu Xuejun

This edition published in 2011
by Singing Dragon
an imprint of Jessica Kingsley Publishers
in co-operation with People's Military Medical Press
116 Pentonville Road
London N1 9JB, UK
and
400 Market Street, Suite 400
Philadelphia, PA 19106, USA

www.singingdragon.com

First published in 2009
by People's Military Medical Press

Copyright © People's Military Medical Press 2009 and 2011

Library of Congress Cataloging in Publication Data
A CIP catalog record for this book is available from the Library of Congress

British Library Cataloguing in Publication Data
A CIP catalogue record for this book is available from the British Library

ISBN 978 1 84819 061 0

Printed and bound in Great Britain
by the MPG Books Group

Contents

About the Authors

Cui Chengbin has rich experience in the treatment of difficult diseases, currently working in the Acupuncture Hospital of China Academy of Chinese Medical Sciences, and lecturing at the Training Center of China Academy of Chinese Medical Sciences. He has led or participated in seven research projects, all of which have been organized by either the World Health Organization or the State Administration of Traditional Chinese Medicine. He has also published many articles in the core journals on the practice and research of Chinese acupuncture and moxibustion, and is the chief editor of four books on acupuncture.

Xing Xiaomin graduated from Shandong University of Traditional Chinese Medicine Acupuncture Department, and is now the deputy director of the rehabilitation department and part-time lecturer at the Hospital of Taishan Medical College. He is a member of both the Shandong Traditional Chinese Medicine and Acupuncture Pain Research Standing Committee, and the Shandong Province Association of Integrative Medicine and Healing Committee. He has 15 years of clinical experience and proficiency in the use of acupuncture, moxibustion and other methods to treat subjects of clinical disease. His publications have featured in the core journals, *Chinese Acupuncture & Moxibustion*, and *Chinese Journal of Clinical Rehabilitation*. He has written more than ten articles, edited four books, and participated in numerous research projects at all levels.

Summary

The contributors to this book are all experts in acupuncture, moxibustion, and Tuina massage, with rich experience in both theory and clinical practice. They view the pathogenesis of migraine from the perspective of both Chinese medicine and Western medicine, introduce the treatments of acupuncture, moxibustion, and Tuina massage, with a selection of case studies to deepen readers' understanding for clinical purposes, and, finally, sum up their own insights gained from practical experience. This book includes detail in a balanced combination of figures and texts, and sets out profound knowledge in a simple way that can easily be put into practise. This is a valuable book for practitioners treating migraine with acupuncture, moxibustion, and Tuina massage.

This book can be utilized for reference by students majoring in acupuncture and moxibustion, and by acupuncture practitioners, patients suffering from migraine, and anyone who is interested in acupuncture and moxibustion.

Foreword

Chinese medicine has an extensive history regarding the treatment of headache. Written during the Period of Spring and Autumn and Warring States, *Huangdi Neijing* has many references to headache. For example, in *Miraculous Pivot: Introduction to Meridians*, it states that dysfunction of the Bladder Meridian manifests as headache, proptosis, and neck stiffness, and in *Plain Questions: Discussion on Various Relationships Concerning the Five Zang Organs*, it is recorded that pain in the vertex is marked by deficiency in the lower and excess in the upper, due to the disorder of the meridians of Foot-Shaoyang and Foot-Taiyang; if it is severe, the disease will be transmitted to the kidneys.

The term "migraine" didn't appear until the Jin and Yuan dynasties. In the book *Ten Texts of Dongyuan: Differentiation of Internal and External Damages* (*Dongyuan Shishu*), it is recorded that the hemispherical headache is called migraine. In addition, in the book *Confucians' Duties to Their Parents* (*Rumen Shiqin*), it is stated that pain in the frontal corner or the part superior to the ear is called migraine.

For the treatment of migraine, much valuable experience has been accumulated by generation after generation of doctors. According to Volume 9 of the book *The Systematic Classic of Acupuncture and Moxibustion* (*Zhenjiu Jiayi Jing*), severe migraine with temporal pulsation can be treated with bloodletting methods and acupuncture in the Gallbladder Meridian of Foot-Shaoyang. In *Odes of Jade Dragon* (*Yulong Ge*), it is recorded that the simultaneous manipulation of two points from SJ-23 Sizhukong to GB-8 Shuaigu can be applied for general headache or migraine, which are not easy to treat. In *Odes of Various Symptoms* (*Baizheng Fu*), it is said that headache can be treated with DU-22 Xinhui and BL-9 Yuzhen; migraine can be treated with GB 5 Xuanlu and GB-4 Hanyan; and severe headache can be treated with DU-18 Qiangjian and ST-40 Fenglong. In *Odes of Xihong* (*Xihong Fu*), it is said that LU-7 Lieque can treat both general and lateral headache; strong reducing manipulation for LU-9 Taiyuan is very effective for headache. Hitherto, many other therapies, such as ear acupuncture, scapula acupuncture, and wrist–ankle acupuncture have been used to treat migraine, and made a contribution to acupuncture, treatment for migraine.

Acupuncture treatment for migraine can achieve an instant and obvious effect, which is why the World Health Organization places migraine into the category of diseases successfully treated by acupuncture.

Migraine is a common disease, which has a close relationship with the endocrine system, food, genetics, and psychological factors. It can lead to dysfunction of the inner or outer nerves and blood vessels of the brain, which impacts on people's work and daily life. Western medication, tranquilizers, and analgesics are used, but have numerous side-effects. However, acupuncture, as a natural therapy, treats migraine well, without these side-effects. Acupuncture is widely accepted among the people.

Dr. Cui Chengbin, Dr. Xing Xiaomin, and their fellow contributors have written this book, *Illustrated Treatment for Migraine Using Acupuncture, Moxibustion and Tuina Massage*, based upon their collected clinical experience. The book introduces both Traditional Chinese Medicine and Western Medicine pathogenesis of migraine, traditional and modern therapies, and some typical case studies, which can deepen readers' understanding of migraine. Their own experience is also demonstrated in the final part of the book.

As the spectrum of disease expands, medical treatments continue to develop. This book provides extensive knowledge for the treatment of migraine, and it is my hope it will bring increased relief to people suffering with migraine.

Professor Wu Zhongchao
Acupuncture Institute, China Academy of Chinese Medical Sciences
Acupuncture Hospital, China Academy of Chinese Medical Sciences
Member of Health Consultation Group for Central Government Leaders

Chapter *1*

Introduction to Migraine

Migraine is a unilateral or bilateral pulsatile headache with periodic and recurrent attacks. Premonitory symptoms, including visual disturbance, such as photophobia, visual field defect, photopsia, and sensory disorders of the face and limbs, often occur before the attack. During the attack, severe headache will take from minutes to hours to peak. It usually involves the temporal area, first, and then spreads to the occipital region, vertex, orbit, and even to the face, neck, or shoulders. The headache starts as a dull pain and develops into a vascular, pulsatile headache, stabbing pain, or sharp pain. It is usually associated with gastrointestinal symptoms, such as nausea, vomiting, and diarrhea, and visual or auditory symptoms. There are sequelae after the attack, such as continuous headache, fatigue, somnolence, and gastrointestinal symptoms. Patients who suffer migraine attacks will function normally during intermittent periods. Research shows that migraine can be divided into several types, and clinically it is seen in terms of composite types, rather than a single type.

Migraine is a kind of neurovascular disease with incidence ranging from 3.7–13.5 percent. It accounts for a quarter of headache patients, and is on the increase. Females account for 60–70 percent of all migraine patients, which is 2–4 times the incidence in males. It can occur at any age but is more common in the age group between 25 and 45 years internationally, and between 20 and 45 years in China. The incidence of migraine is highest in European people, followed by African people, while the lowest incidence is for Asian people. Frequency of attack varies among individuals, with fixed or diverse attack cycles. According to one survey, the average frequency of migraine attacks is 1.5 per month. At least 10 percent of migraine patients will suffer one attack per week.

Clinical manifestations

The clinical manifestations of migraine are as follows: periodic, recurrent attacks of lateral or bilateral pulsatile headache, in which the property and process of each attack are similar. There are many associated premonitory symptoms, such as visual symptoms, dysfunction of the motor system, and emotional changes. During the attack, patients will suffer from severe headache and other symptoms of the central nervous system and autonomic nervous system; they will perform normally in the intermittent period between attacks. The attack frequency will vary from individual to individual; somebody with a long attack period may have only a few attacks in his or her whole lifetime, while someone with a short attack period may have several attacks in a day. Some people experience regular attacks (for example, female patients' attack period may correspond with the menstrual period), while other attacks are irregular and the headache may not recur for a long time, for no evident reason, following one or several attacks. According to statistics, patients will suffer 1.5 attacks on average, and at least 10 percent of migraine patients will suffer one attack per week. The attack may be induced by seasonal transition, for example from autumn to winter, or from winter to spring. Headache often occurs in the daytime, and sometimes at night.

PHASES OF A MIGRAINE

A migraine attack has three distinct stages: the prodromal phase, the attack phase, and the post-headache phase.

Prodromal phase

About 10 percent of patients will have premonitory symptoms, which are caused by spasm of cerebral vessels. Local ischemia caused by spasm of blood vessels provokes these symptoms in different parts of the body. Because contraction of the internal carotid artery occurs at an early stage, symptoms of visual disturbance arise, mainly among children, on the opposite side to the occurring headache. They will experience visual sensations of flashing and dots, which are associated with photophobia, and sometimes have tunnel vision, unilateral blindness, transient vision loss, visual disturbance, metamorphopsia, polyopia, diplopia, and altered color vision. Patients may, in addition, experience dizziness, pallor, general malaise, speech disorder, numbness of face or limbs, and premonitory symptoms of movement disorder, such as facial paralysis, or hemiparalysis. The premonitory symptoms will last from several minutes to half an hour, and then gradually disappear as the patient enters the headache phase.

Attack phase

Patients can either go straight into the headache phase, or following the prodromal phase; sometimes migraine occurs in the prodromal phase. In the attack stage, reactive dilation due to spasm of the intracranial and extracranial arteries leads to intracranial congestion due to high perfusion, which causes migraine. The headache often attacks unilaterally, and sometimes transfers to the other side, or it may occur bilaterally. It is located in the temporal and frontal regions, or extends to the occipital region, nape, vertex, and orbit, and sometimes radiates to the face or shoulders. Mild migraine will manifest first as dull pain, and transform into vascular, pulsatile pain. It may spread gradually, or manifest as stabbing pain, sharp pain, tension, and throbbing, pain around the orbit or deep in the eyeball, or an icy feeling around the orbit or temporal region. Some patients may feel irritable, overly excited, or have a sensation of emptiness in the head.

A migraine attack will be associated with gastrointestinal symptoms, such as vomiting, nausea, or diarrhea, which occur a few minutes after the headache. In addition, other accompanying symptoms include syncope, altered states of consciousness, mood alteration, speech disorder, memory impairment, dizziness, ataxia, rapid breathing, high fever, pallor, pupillary abnormalities, ophthalmoplegia, olfactory hallucination, tinnitus, nasal obstruction, and increased nasal secretion.

A typical migraine will become aggravated after onset, and reach its peak within several minutes or up to half an hour. It may last between several hours and several days, and then weaken gradually to enter the post-headache phase.

Post-headache phase

In this stage, the symptoms are mainly headache of sequelae, or other uncomfortable feelings, and associated with tiredness and drowsiness. The headache will disappear gradually and transform into sleep, which is the end of the attack.

COMMON TYPES OF MIGRAINE

Symptoms of migraine are complicated; for example, the same patient may manifest with different symptoms during each attack. Due to lack of a gold standard, the diagnosis of migraine depends on detailed investigation and long-term follow-up.

Migraine is divided into three types by the International Headache Society: common migraine, classic migraine, and specific migraine. The common migraine (migraine without aura) accounts for 80 percent of all migraines, and classic migraine (migraine with aura) is 15 percent of all migraines; both are common in clinic.

Common migraine

Factors such as tiredness, menstruation, nervousness, hot weather, alcohol, taking a shower, fever, and even over-sleeping at the weekend will induce migraine. A common migraine is not preceded by an aura, with pain from moderate to severe. It occurs on one or both sides of the head, and possibly the whole head, and is less severe than classic migraine. The migraine lasts from several hours to several days with intermittent phase.

DIAGNOSTIC CRITERTIA OF COMMON MIGRAINE

- More than five attacks.
- Headache lasts from four to 72 hours; for children under 15, it lasts from two to 48 hours.
- The headache has more than two of the following features:
    o attack on one side only
    o pulsatile pain
    o moderate to severe in intensity (daily activities limited)
    o made worse by normal physical activity, such as going upstairs.
- Accompanied by one of the following symptoms:
    o nausea and/or vomiting
    o sensitivity to light and sound.
- Other factors for headache excluded.
- No abnormal medical history and no somatic diseases.
- No other similar diseases.

Classic migraine

The main feature of classic migraine is an aura preceding the headache.

DIAGNOSTIC CRITERIA OF CLASSIC MIGRAINE

- More than two attacks.
- At least three of the following four symptoms:
    o one or more premonitory symptoms which can be completely reversed, indicating local dysfunction of the cerebrum or brain stem

○ at least one premonitory symptom develops gradually, and lasts for more than four minutes (usually from five to 20 minutes); or two premonitory symptoms occurring one at a time

○ premonitory symptoms last for less than 60 minutes (if there is more than one premonitory symptom, duration will increase)

○ there is no intermittent phase between aura and headache: headache, vomiting and/or photophobia occur after aura; the intermittent phase is less than 60 minutes; headache usually lasts from four to 72 hours (headache can occur before or together with aura).

• Matches at least one of the following criteria, to exclude headache resulting from other causes:

○ no organic diseases revealed in medical history and clinical examination

○ appears to have organic disease according to illness history and clinical exam, but this is ruled out by laboratory test

○ has organic disease, unrelated to first onset of migraine.

Specific types of migraine

There are several types of migraines which are rare in clinic, such as ophthalmoplegic migraine, migraine with hemiparalysis, basal-type migraine, and retinal migraine. It is essential to make the correct diagnosis.

Ophthalmoplegic migraine: First onset of the migraine is before 12 years old; the pain is located on or around the orbit and radiates to the lateral side of the face. Ophthalmoplegia manifests as blepharoptosis of the affected side, pupil dilation, double vision, and restricted movement of the eyeball upwards and downwards, and abduction. Recurrent attacks will lead to permanent paralysis. Ophthalmoplegia associated with the headache will continue, even after the headache has been relieved.

Migraine with hemiparalysis: Hemiparalysis is the aura of migraine, which manifests as decreased power and the sensation in all four limbs, accompanied by joint disorder, aphasia, tremor, nystagmus, retinal degeneration, deafness, and ataxia. Hemiparalysis attacks usually start in childhood and end at adolescence, with transformation to other types of migraine.

Basal-type migraine: It often affects adolescent females (correlating with a menstrual period), most of whom have a family history. The mechanism is dysfunction of brain stem nerves, which leads to sensitivity to light, hallucination, and even blindness; other symptoms include dizziness, joint disorder, aphasia, tinnitus, ataxia, transient memory, numbness of limbs and perioral lips, mental instability.

Retinal migraine: Visual field defect with spots, lasting for about 60 minutes; headache will appear either within about 60 minutes following onset of visual symptoms, or before onset. During the intermittent period, ophthalmic examination is negative, to rule out cerebral thrombosis.

DIFFERENTIAL DIAGNOSIS

Headache is divided into primary and secondary groups. Migraine belongs to the primary group, which also includes tension-type headache, cluster headache, and trigeminal neurogenic headache. These four types together account for 90 percent of all headaches. Patients with the complaint of headache should receive differential diagnosis.

Differential diagnosis of primary headache

Tension-type headache: Also called muscular contractive headache, it manifests as oppression, with heaviness of the head due to continuous contraction of muscle in the head and neck, and is the most common type of headache. Patients have tenderness and stiffness in the neck, scapula area, and back.

Cluster headache: Often confined to one side, with headaches occuring in a short-term, frequent attack peaking every 10–15 minutes, and lasting for about one hour. It is unbearable but relived relatively quickly. The pain is stabbing, sharp, and associated with sympathetic nerve symptoms of the face and nose.

Trigeminal neurogenic headache: Similar to cluster headache, with the pain mainly confined to the temporal region and around the orbit. The severe pain lasts only for a short time with high frequency of attacks (from a few to hundreds of attacks). It is often accompanied by conjunctival congestion, lacrimation, nasal obstruction, runny nose, frontal sweating, contracted pupil, and ptosis.

Differential diagnosis of secondary headache

Migraine accompanied by signals from the nervous system is probably caused by organic disease, so the diagnosis should be made using general physical examination, neurological examination, and laboratory examination such as blood test, cerebrospinal fluid test, ultrasound of the nervous system, X-ray, cranial CT, MRI, MRA, and EEG. There are several conditions that may be indicated by differential diagnosis, as follows:

- **Headache due to trauma of the head and neck:** Headache due to cerebral concussion.

- **Headache due to vascular disease of the head and neck:** Intracranial aneurysm; cerebral vascular malformation; subarachnoid hemorrhage;

cerebral hemorrhage; cerebral ischemia; temporal arteritis and hypertension, etc.

- **Headache due to non-cerebrovascular diseases:** Headache due to increase or decrease in intracranial pressure, intracranial tumor, and non-vascular inflammation such as meningitis, etc.

- **Headache due to psychiatric disease:** The occurrence and severity of headaches bears a close relationship to mental status. Headache is often associated with insomnia, distractibility, poor memory, dizziness, and irritability.

- **Headache due to infection or abnormal metabolism:** All febrile disease and general infection can lead to headache. Alcohol and drug abuse can also induce headache. Pain may be relieved by decrease in body temperature.

Chinese medicine diagnosis

CLINICAL DIAGNOSTIC CRITERIA

- Headache affects the frontal region, temporal region, vertex, and even the whole head.

- The quality of the headache is beating pain, stabbing pain, distending pain, dull pain, or severe, unbearable pain.

- The attack will last from minutes to hours, or days to weeks.

- It occurs without any indication and gradually becomes severe, or there are recurrent attacks.

- The etiology of the headache should be detected by blood test, hypertension; cerebrospinal fluid test and EEG if necessary, or even transcranial doppler ultrasound, CT, and MRI, to exclude organic diseases.

ZANG-FU DIFFERENTIATION

According to experts' clinical experience, the syndromes of blood stasis, phlegm dampness, and hyperactivity of liver yang are the main factors. Others include liver stagnation, liver fire, wind cold, wind heat, wind damp, and blood deficiency. Based on clinical study, Zang-Fu differentiation includes five syndromes.

1. Syndrome of hyperactivity of liver yang

- **Major symptoms:** Headache with distension; irritability; red eyes and bitter taste.

- **Minor symptoms:** Ruddy complexion; dry mouth; red tongue; yellow tongue coating; (rapid) wiry pulse.

2. Syndrome of phlegm turbidity

- **Major symptoms:** Headache with property of heaviness; chest distension; vomiting or nausea with phlegm or excess saliva.

- **Minor symptoms:** Bland taste in mouth; poor appetite; enlarged tongue; white, greasy tongue coating; wiry/slippery pulse.

3. Syndrome of kidney deficiency

- **Major symptoms:** Headache with feeling of emptiness; dizziness; soreness/tiredness of waist and knee, five center heat.

- **Minor symptoms:** Fatigue; tinnitus; red tongue with sparse tongue coating; deep, weak pulse.

4. Syndrome of blood stasis

- **Major symptoms:** Headache with stabbing quality and confined location.

- **Minor symptoms:** Dark purple tongue with ecchymosis; white, thin tongue coating; deep, thready pulse, or thready and rough pulse.

5. Syndrome of qi and blood deficiency

- **Major symptoms:** Recurrent headache with property of dull pain, aggravated by tiredness.

- **Minor symptoms:** Palpitation; poor appetite; spontaneous sweating; fatigue; pale complexion; pale tongue; white, thready tongue coating; deep, thready, weak pulse.

MERIDIAN DIFFERENTIATION

Syndrome differentiation using the meridians is considered secondary to Zang-Fu differentiation, although these methods are closely related to each other. Zang-Fu differentiation focuses on Zang-Fu organ dysfunction, which leads to various symptoms; while syndrome differentiation by meridians focuses on abnormal reactions relating to the relevant meridian course.

- **Symptoms related to the Shaoyang Meridian:** Unilateral or bilateral headache confined to the region around the outer canthus; bitter tastes; sighing; poor complexion; discomfort in the ears, throat, cheek, and lateral side of the body; thoracic and hypochondriac pain. (Shaoyang Sanjiao Meridian of Hand connects with the ear, and runs to outer canthus; Shaoyang Gallbladder Meridian of Foot originates from outer canthus, and runs to hairline corner, the branch reaches posterior to outer canthus.)

- **Symptoms related to the Jueyin Meridian:** Palpitation; chest distension; poor mood, five center heat, etc. (Jueyin Liver Meridian of Foot goes out from the frontal head, connects with Governor Channel at the vertex.)

- **Symptoms related to the Yangming Meridian:** Headache is confined to one or both sides of the frontal region of the head; associated with vomiting, dysfunction of gastrointestinal system. (Yangming Stomach Meridian of Foot originates from the nose, reaches the nasal root, goes along the hairline, to reach frontal head.)

- **Symptoms related to the Taiyang Meridian:** Headache is in the occipital region and extends to nape. Eye pain with lacrimation; nasal obstruction; nasal bleeding, etc. (Taiyang Bladder Meridian of Foot originates from inner canthus, reaching the frontal region of the head; the branch from vertex reaches the tip of ear; the main branch goes into brain, then goes downward along the nape.)

- **Symptoms related to the Governor Channel:** Headache around the midline of the head, connects with nape, accompanied with fever; abnormal mental state. (Governor Channel flows along the spinal cord, to DU-16 Fengfu, reaches the vertex, goes across frontal head and to the nose.)

Chapter 2

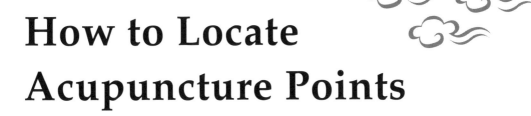

How to Locate Acupuncture Points

Section I Fundamentals for Point Location

Acupuncture points are specific sites through which qi and blood of Zang-Fu organs and meridians is transported to the surface of the body. Points are classified into three categories: points of the 14 meridians, Extraordinary points, and Ashi points.

The *points of the 14 meridians* include those distributed on the 12 regular meridians, as well as two of the extraoridinary meridians – the Conception Vessel and Governor Vessel. There are six other extraordinary meridians, which have a close relationship with these 14 meridians. The points provide not only the pathological manifestation of the related meridian and organs, but also the location for acupuncture treatment.

Although not listed in the system of 14 meridians, *Extraordinary points* have their name and location, and they are useful in therapy with a special function to treat certain diseases.

Ashi points are tender spots or sensitive spots present in certain areas of the body. They are often proximal or distal to the disease location.

Rules for point indication

Rules for point indication are divided into two categories: *proximal effect* and *distal effect*.

Proximal effect is a common feature of all points, as each point can treat the disease of organs near to it, or disease at the point location. In the treatment of migraine, major points are chosen from the head, in order to utilize the point's proximal effect. The points comprise those in the Shaoyang Meridian (such as SJ-23 Sizhukong, GB-8 Shuaigu, GB-20 Fengchi, GB-5 Xuanlu and GB-4 Heyan, etc.); in the Taiyang Meridian (such as BL-2 Cuanzu, BL-10 Tianzhu, BL-9 Yuzhen, etc.); in the Yangming Meridian (such as ST-8 Touwei, etc.) and in the Governor Channel (such as DU-20 Baihui, DU-21 Qianding, DU-19 Houding, etc.). Points such as BL-1 Jingming, ST-1 Chengqi, and ST-2 Sibai can be added to treat migraine with visual premonitory symptoms, or ophthalmoplegic migraine. SI-19 Tinggong and GB-2 Tinghui can be added to treat migraine associated with hearing disorder.

Distal effect is the basic rule for indication of points of the 14 meridians. The points of 14 meridians, especially points of the 12 regular meridians, which are below the knees and elbows, can treat not only disease of regional parts, but also diseases related to the proximal part of organs connected with the meridians, and even the systemic diseases.

For the treatment of migraine, besides the points in the head, some points in the four limbs will be applied, including the points of the Shaoyang Meridian (such as GB-41 Zulinqi, GB-40 Qiuxu, GB-34 Yanglingquan, SJ-3 Zhongzhu, and SJ-2 Yemen, etc.); the points of the Taiyang Meridian (such as BL-60 Kunlun, BL-67 Zhiyin and SI-3 Houxi, etc.); and LI-4 Hegu in the Yangming Meridian. Some other points will be added as the adjunct point or according to syndrome differentiation such as ST-36 Zusanli and ST-40 Fenglong.

Application of specific points

Among the points of the 14 meridians, some have specific properties, and are grouped together under special names.

THE FIVE SHU POINTS

Along each of the 12 regular meridians, below the elbow or knee, lie five specific points, namely Jing-well, Ying-spring, Shu-stream, Jing-river, and He-sea (see Table 2.1 and 2.2). The five Shu points start from the extremities of the limbs as far as the knee (or elbow) in the order of Jing-well, Ying-spring, Shu-stream, Jing-river, and He-sea. In *Miraculous Pivot: Healthy Human Energy by the Day and Night Corresponds with the Energies of the Four Seasons*, it is recorded that:

- Jing-well points can treat visceral disease.

- Ying-spring points can treat diseases with complexion change.

- Shu-stream points can treat chronic disease.

- Jing-river points can treat disease with voice change.

- He-sea points can treat disease with hemorrhage, gastric disease, or disease due to improper diet.

Table 2.1 Correspondence between the points of the six yin meridians of the hand and foot and the Five Elements

Meridian	Jing-well (Wood)	Ying-spring (Fire)	Shu-stream (Earth)	Jing-river (Metal)	He-sea (Water)
Taiyin Lung Meridian of the Hand	LU-11 Shaoshang	LU-10 Yuji	LU-9 Taiyuan	LU-8 Jingqu	LU-5 Chize
Jueyin Pericardium Meridian of the Hand	PC-9 Zhongchong	PC-8 Laogong	PC-7 Daling	PC-5 Jianshi	PC-3 Quze
Shaoyin Heat Meridian of the Hand	HT-9 Shaochong	HT-8 Shaofu	HT-7 Shenmen	HT-4 Lingdao	HT-3 Shaohai
Taiyin Spleen Meridian of the Foot	SP-1 Yinbai	SP-2 Dadu	SP-3 Taibai	SP-5 Shangqiu	SP-9 Yinlingquan
Jueyin Liver Meridian of the Foot	LR-1 Dadun	LR-2 Xingjian	LR-3 Taichong	LR-4 Zhongfeng	LR-8 Ququan
Shaoyin Kidney Meridian of the Foot	KI-1 Yongquan	KI-2 Rangu	KI-3 Taixi	KI-7 Fuliu	KI-10 Yingu

Table 2.2 Correspondence between the points of the six yang meridians of the hand and foot and the Five Elements

Meridian	Jing-well (Metal)	Ying-spring (Water)	Shu-stream (Earth)	Yuan-source	Jing-river (Fire)	He-sea (Earth)
Yangming Large Intestine Meridian of the Hand	LI-1 Shangyang	LI-2 Erjian	LI-3 Sanjian	LI-4 Hegu	LI-5 Yangxi	LI-11 Quchi
Shaoyang Sanjiao Meridian of the Hand	SJ-1 Guanchong	SJ-2 Yemen	SJ-3 Zhongzhu	SJ-4 Yangchi	SJ-6 Zhigou	SJ-10 Tianjing
Taiyan Small Intestine Meridian of the Hand	SI-1 Shaoze	SI-2 Qiangu	SI-3 Houxi	SI-4 Wangu	SI-5 Yanggu	SI-8 Xiaohai
Yangming Stomach Meridian of the Foot	ST-45 Lidui	ST-44 Neiting	ST-43 Xiangu	ST-42 Chongyang	ST-41 Jiexi	ST-36 Zusanli
Shaoyang Gallbladder Meridian of the Foot	GB-44 Zuqiaoyin	GB-43 Xiaxi	GB-41 Zulinqi	GB-40 Qiuxu	GB-38 Yangfu	GB-34 Yanglingquan
Taiyang Bladder Meridian of the Foot	BL-67 Zhiyin	BL-66 Zutonggu	BL-65 Sugu	BL-64 Jinggu	BL-60 Kunlun	BL-40 Weizhong

THE BACK-SHU POINTS AND FRONT-MU POINTS

Back-Shu points are the points at the back where the qi of the respective Zang-Fu organs is infused. Front-Mu points are those points on the chest and abdomen where the qi of the respective Zang-Fu organs is infused (Table 2.3). Both groups are located on the trunk, which indicates their close relationship with the Zang-Fu organs. In the clinic, they can be used in combination to treat diseases of the Zang-Fu organs, and they can also applied respectively to treat the dysfunction of organs connected with the corresponding meridians. For example, since the liver opens into the eyes, BL-18 Ganshu is used to treat eye disease; since the kidney opens into the ears, deafness can be treated with BL-23 Shenhu.

Table 2.3 Back-Shu points and Front-Mu points of the Zang-Fu organs

Back-Shu points and Front-Mu points of the five Zang organs		
Front-Mu	**Zang organ**	**Back-Shu**
LU-1 Zhongfu	Lung	BL-13 Feishu
RN-17 Danzhong	Pericardium	BL-14 Jueyinshu
RN-14 Juque	Heart	BL-15 Xinshu
LR-14 Qimen	Liver	BL-18 Ganshu
LR-13 Zhangmen	Spleen	BL-20 Pishu
GB-25 Jingmen	Kidney	BL-23 Shenshu
Back-Shu points and Front-Mu points of the six Fu organs		
Front-Mu	**Fu organ**	**Back-Shu**
RN-12 Zhongwan	Stomach	BL-21 Weishu
GB-24 Riyue	Gallbladder	BL-19 Danshu
RN-3 Zhongji	Bladder	BL-28 Pangguangshu
ST-25 Tianshu	Large intestine	BL-25 Dachangshu
RN-5 Shimen	Sanjiao	BL-22 Sanjiaoshu
RN-4 Guanyuan	Small intestine	BL-27 Xiaochangshu

In the treatment of migraine, Back-Shu points and Front-Mu points will be applied according to the particular syndrome; for example, Back-Shu points of the liver, gallbladder, kidney, heart, and spleen will be used to regulate the corresponding organs; Front-Mu points such as RN-12 Zhongwan, RN-17 Tanzhong, RN-4 Guanyuan, and BL-17 Geshu will be used with the aim of regulating qi movement, dispersing phlegm, and enhancing blood circulation.

THE YUAN-SOURCE POINTS AND THE LUO-CONNECTING POINTS

A Yuan-source point is a site where the qi of the Zang-Fu organs is retained. Each of the 12 regular meridians has a Yuan-source point near the knee or elbow

– points called the 12 Yuan-source points in the classics of Chinese medicine (Table 2.4). "If the five Zang-organs or the six Fu organs have diseases, the corresponding Yuan-source points should be applied." In the six yang meridians, the Yuan-source points are independent ones located behind the Shu-stream points, while in the six yin meridians, the Yuan-source points are also the Shu-stream points.

Each of the 12 regular meridians also has a collateral in the extremities connecting a definite pair of yin and yang meridians which are externally–internally related. Each of the 12 collaterals has a Luo-connecting point, below the knee (or elbow) of each of the four limbs. Together with RN-15 Jiuwei (the Luo-connecting point of the Conception Channel, located in the abdomen), DU-1 Changqiang (the Luo-connecting point of the Governor Channel, located in the sacrococcygeal region), and SP-21 Dabao (the Luo-connecting point of the Spleen Meridian, located in the costal region), they are called the 15 Lu points (Table 2.4).

Table 2.4 Yuan-source points and Luo-connecting points of the 12 meridians

Meridian	Yuan-source points	Luo-connecting points
Taiyin Lung Meridian of the Hand	LU-9 Taixi	LU-7 Lieque
Jueyin Pericardium Meridian of the Hand	PC-7 Daling	PC-6 Neiguan
Shaoyin Heart Meridian of the Hand	HT-7 Shenmen	HT-5 Tongli
Taiyin Spleen Meridian of the Foot	SP-3 Taibai	SP-4 Gongsun
Jueyin Liver Meridian of the Foot	LI-3 Taichong	LR-5 Ligou
Shaoyin Kidney Meridian of the Foot	KI-3 Taixi	KI-4 Dazhong
Yangming Large Intestine Meridian of the Hand	LI-4 Hegu	LI-5 Pianli
Shaoyang Sanjiao Meridian of the Hand	SJ-4 Yangchi	SJ-5 Waiguan
Taiyang Small Intestine Meridian of the Hand	SI-4 Wangu	SI-7 Zhizheng
Yangming Stomach Meridian of the Foot	ST-42 Chongyang	ST-40 Fenglong
Shaoyang Gallbladder Meridian of the Foot	GB-40 Qiuxu	GB-37 Guangming
Taiyang Bladder Meridian of the Foot	BL-64 Jinggu	BL-58 Feiyang

Yuan-source points and Luo-connecting points can be applied separately or in combination. The organs initially involved will be treated with the Yuan-source point of the corresponding meridian, while the ones affected later will be treated with the Luo-connecting points of the corresponding meridian.

In the treatment of migraine, both Yuan-source points and Luo-connecting points will be applied frequently, with combinations of the two for qi regulation of exterior–interior meridians. For example, LI-4 Hegu and LU-7 Lieque will be used together to move qi, invigorate blood, open orifices, and dispel phlegm.

THE XI-CLEFT POINTS

"Cleft" means a natural crack in something. A Xi-cleft point is a site where the qi of the meridian is deeply converged. There is a Xi-cleft point in each of the 12 regular channels, in the extremities, below the knee and elbow, and one in each of the four extra meridians (Yin Link Channel, Yang Link Channel, Yin Heel Channel, Yang Heel Channel) – 16 in all (see Table 2.5). The Xi-cleft points are used in treating acute disorders in the areas supplied by their corresponding meridians, and disorders in their respectively related Zang-Fu organs. Xi-cleft points of the yin meridians will be used for blood syndrome, while those of the yang meridians will be used for pain.

Table 2.5 The 16 Xi-cleft points

Meridian	Xi-cleft point	Meridian	Xi-cleft point
Taiyin Lung Meridian of the Hand	LU-7 Kongzui	Shaoyin Kidney Meridian of the Foot	KI-5 Shuiquan
Jueyin Pericardium of the Hand	PC-4 Ximen	Yangming Stomach Meridian of the Foot	ST-34 Liangqiu
Shaoyin Heart Meridian of the Hand	HT-6 Yinxi	Shaoyang Gallbladder Meridian of the Foot	GB-36 Waiqiu
Yangming Large Intestine Meridian of the Hand	LI-7 Wenliu	Taiyang Bladder Meridian of the Foot	BL-63 Jinmen
Shaoyang Sanjiao Meridian of the Hand	SJ-7 Huizong	Yin Link Channel	KI-9 Zhubin
Taiyang Small Intestine Meridian of the Hand	SI-6 Yanglao	Yang Link Channel	GB-35 Yangjiao
Taiyin Spleen Meridian of the Foot	SP-8 Diji	Yin Heel Channel	KI-80 Jiaoxin
Jueyin Liver Meridian of the Foot	LR-6 Zhongdu	Yang Heel Channel	BL-59 Fuyang

In the treatment of migraine, Xi-cleft points in yang meridians are used frequently, such as GB-35 Yangjiao, Xi-cleft of Yang Link Channel; BL-59 Fuyang, Xi-cleft of Yang Heel Channel; BL-63 Jinmen, Xi-cleft point of Taiyang Bladder Meridian of Foot; and LI-7 Wenliu, Xi-cleft point of Taiyang Small Intestine Meridian of Hand.

THE LOWER-SEA POINTS

The six points called the Lower-sea points of the six Fu organs are the sites where the qi of the six Fu organs is infused and connects with the three Foot yang meridians (Table 2.6). Located near the knee, the Lower-sea points can have a significant effect on diseases of the six Fu organs. It is recorded in *Miraculous Pivot: The Visceral Diseases Caused by Evil Energy* that Lower-sea points are used to treat disorders of the Fu organs. The appropriate points can be applied, corresponding with the organs affected by evil qi.

Table 2.6 Lower-sea points of the six Fu organs

Taiyang Small Intestine Meridian of the Hand	ST-39 Xiajuxu
Shaoyang Sanjiao Meridian of the Hand	BL-39 Weiyang
Yangming Large Intestine Meridian of the Hand	ST-37 Shangjuxu
Taiyang Bladder Meridian of the Foot	BL-40 Weizhong
Shaoyang Gallbladder Meridian of the Foot	GB-34 Yanglingquan
Yangming Stomach Meridian of the Foot	ST-36 Zusanli

In the treatment of migraine, if the disease relates to dysfunction of the Fu organs, the Lower-sea points can be applied. Migraine due to gastrointestinal dysfunction should be treated with ST-36 Zusanli, ST-37 Shangjuxu and ST-39 Xiajuxu to regulate the function of the gastrointestinal system.

THE EIGHT MEETING POINTS

The eight Meeting points are those where the vital substance of the Zang organs, Fu organs, qi, blood, tendons, vessels, bone, and marrow converge. They are located on the trunk and the four limbs (Table 2.7). Each point can treat disease related to its particular property.

Table 2.7 The eight Meeting points

Zang organs converging point	LV-3 Zhangmen
Fu organs converging point	RN-12 Zhongwan
Qi converging point	RN-17 Tanzhong
Blood converging point	BL-17 Geshu
Tendon converging point	GB-34 Yanglingquan
Vessel converging point	LU-9 Taiyuan
Bone converging point	BL-11 Dazhu
Marrow converging point	GB-39 Juegu / Xuanzhong

In migraine, pathological changes often involve dysfunction of the Zang and Fu organs, imbalance of qi and blood, yin and yang, and malnutrition of tendon, vessel, brain, and marrow. That is why the eight Meeting points are used as supplementary points.

CONFLUENCE POINTS OF THE EIGHT EXTRAORDINARY MERIDIANS

The points are located on the limbs, below the elbow and knee, where the 12 regular meridians communicate with the eight extraordinary meridians (Table 2.8). Clinically, the points can be applied separately, according to their related meridians, and can also be used in combination with points on the head or body, following the principle of far and nearby points-combination. Points can also be chosen according to the principle of upper and lower points-combination.

Table 2.8 Confluence points of the eight extraordinary meridians

Meridian	Points	Extraordinary meridian	Indication (part of the body)
Spleen	SP-4 Gongsun	Chong Channel	Heart, stomach, chest
Pericardium	PC-6 Neiguan	Yin Link Channel	
Gallbladder	GB-41 Zulinqi	Belt Channel	Inner canthus, cheek, neck, shoulder, retroauricular area
Sanjiao	SJ-5 Waiguan	Yang Link Channel	
Small intestine	SI-3 Houxi	Governor Channel	Inner canthus, nape, shoulder, scapular area
Bladder	BL-62 Shenmai	Yang Heel Channel	
Lung	LU-7 Lieque	Conception Channel	Chest, lung, diaphragm, throat
Kidney	KI-6 Zhaohai	Yin Heel Channel	

The eight points have a close relationship with the eight extraordinary meridians, and have therapeutic properties for treating diseases of the extraordinary meridians and their related organs. Since the etiology of migraine is due to pathological changes in the qi and blood of the Governor Channel, Yang Link Channel, and Yang Heel Channel, SJ-5 Waiguan, SI-3 Houxi, BL-62 Shenmai, and GB-41 Zulinqi will be used as supplementary points. The eight points can be applied according to the principle of upper and lower points-combination, which extends these points' indication. For migraine with dysfunction of the gastrointestinal system, SP-4 Gongsong will be used together with PC-6 Neiguan. In this way the eight points can be applied for treatment of migraine according to syndrome differentiation.

CROSSING POINTS

Crossing points are those points at the intersection of two or more channels. They are mainly distributed on the head, face, and trunk, and are indicated in diseases involving several channels. Crossing points are distributed extensively, and in large numbers. For migraine in which the meridian distribution is not clear, the Crossing points can be applied to regulate several meridians simultaneously, thereby using fewer points to relieve patients' pain.

Principle of point selection

SELECTION OF LOCAL POINTS

points can be used to treat diseases on or adjacent to themselves. Depending on their location, points on the head will be selected for the treatment of migraine.

SELECTION OF REMOTE POINTS

points can be used in treating disorders in the remote areas supplied by their pertaining meridians, which are often located below the knee and elbow. In *Plain Questions*: *Major Discussions on the Administration of the Five Emotions* it is said that disease located in the upper part of the body can be cured by treating the lower part of the body, and disease located in the lower part of the body can be cured by treating the upper part of the body. According to the records, points on the extremities, especially the ends of the feet, have a significant effect on migraine.

SELECTIONS OF POINTS ACCORDING TO SYNDROME DIFFERENTIATION

Depending on individual syndrome differentiation (such as syndrome differentiation of the meridians or syndrome differentiation of the Zang-Fu organs), the points will be selected as supplementary. For example, migraine of the Shaoyang or Yangming meridian will be treated with the addition of some points in the corresponding meridian.

Migraine with the syndrome of hyperactivity of liver yang will be treated with BL-23 Shenshu, BL-18 Ganshu, KI-3 Taixi, and LR-3 Taichong to pacify the liver, nourish yin, and subdue yang, while for migraine with the syndrome of collateral stagnation of phlegm and stasis, points including RN-12 Zhongwan, ST-40 Fenglong, BL-17 Geshu, SP-10 Xuehai, and SP-6 Sanyinjiao will be added.

POINTS SELECTION BASED ON CLINICAL EXPERIENCE

According to clinical experience, certain points (such as EX-HN-5 Taiyang, GB-20 Fengchi, and the line linking GB-5 Xuanlu and GB-6 Xuanli, which has special function to headache or migraine) will be applied.

Section II Location of Commonly Used Points

Methods of locating points

Accuracy in locating points will help to achieve good outcome of acupuncture treatment, and the following three methods of locating points are now introduced.

LOCATION OF POINTS BY BONE PROPORTION (CUN)

On the basis of anatomical landmarks, a measuring method has been established for locating points at a certain distance between anatomical landmarks. The width or length of various portions of the human body is divided into definite numbers of equal divisions, each division being termed 1 cun, which are taken as the unit of measurement in locating points. The commonly used standards for proportional measurement are shown in Table 2.9. Figure 2.1 is an illustration of proportional measurement.

Table 2.9 Commonly used standards for proportional measurement

Body part	Origin and termination	Proportional measurement	Longitudinal/ transverse	Instruction
Head	From the anterior hairline to the posterior hairline.	12 cun	Longitudinal measurement	If the anterior hairline is indistinguishable, measurement can be done from the glabella and 3 cun added. So too with the posterior hairline: measurement can be taken from the point of DU-14 Dazhui and 3 cun added. The distance from the glabella to DU-14 Dazhui is 18 cun.
Chest and abdomen	Between the two mastoid processes.	9 cun	Transverse measurement	The distance between the two mastoid processes is 9 cun measured transversely.
	From RN-22 Tiantu to the sternocostal angle.	9 cun	Longitudinal measurement	The chest and costal region will be measured longitudinally, based on the width of rib. Each rib is about 1.6 cun in width.
	From the sternocostal angle to the center of the umbilicus.	8 cun		
	From the center of the umbilicus to the upper border of the symphysis pubis.	5 cun		
	Between the two nipples.	8 cun	Transverse measurement	For the female, the two midline clavicular lines will be used, the distance between which is also 8 cun.
Back	From the vertebra magna to the coccygeal vertebra.	21 vertebrae	Longitudinal measurement	Points on the back are located corresponding to the vertebrae. Clinically, the inferior angle of the scapula is level with the seventh thoracic vertebra; the iliac crest is level with the sixteenth vertebra (fourth lumbar vertebra).
	Between the medial borders of the scapulae	6 cun	Transverse measurement	

cont.

Table 2.9 Commonly used standards for proportional measurement *cont.*

Body part	Origin and termination	Proportional measurement	Longitudinal/ transverse	Instruction
Upper limb	From the end of the axillary fold to the transverse cubital crease.	9 cun	Longitudinal measurement	These proportional measurement are used for the three Hand yang meridians and the three Hand yin meridians.
	From the transverse cubital crease to the transverse carpal crease.	12 cun		
Lateral side of chest	From the axillary fossa to the end of the 11th rib.	12 cun	Longitudinal measurement	The eleventh rib is a floating rib.
Lateral side of the abdomen	From the 11th rib to the greater trochanter of the femur.	9 cun	Longitudinal measurement	
Lower limb	From the level of the upper border of the symphysis pubis to the medial epicondyle of the femur.	18 cun	Longitudinal measurement	From the great trochanter of the femur to the middle of the patella.
	From the lower border of the medial condyle of the tibia to the tip of the medial malleolus.	13 cun		
	From the transverse crease of hip to the middle of the patella.	14 cun		
	From the center of the patella to the tip of the lateral malleolus.	16 cun		
	From the tip of the lateral maleolus to the plantar surface of the foot.	3 cun		

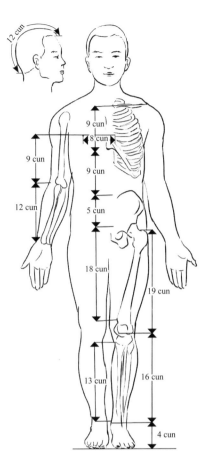

Figure 2.1 Illustration of proportional measurement

ACCORDING TO ANATOMICAL LANDMARKS

Anatomical landmarks on the surface of the body are of specific significance in locating points. If the sites of points are in the vicinity of, or on, such landmarks, they can be located directly. The landmarks are divided into two categories: immovable and movable landmarks.

Immovable marks

Prominence or depression of the bones or muscles, eyes, mouth, hairline, nails, nipple, umbilicus, etc. will be easily detected when the body is relaxed, and can be used for locating points. For example:

- GB-34 Yanglingquan is located at 1 cun anterior and posterior to the fibula head.

- SP-6 Sanyinjiao is 3 cun above the tip of the medial malleolus and on the posterior border of the tibia.

- BL-2 Cuanzu is on the medial end of the eyebrow.

- ST-25 Tianshu is 2 cun lateral to umbilicus.

Movable marks

Fissures, depressions, wrinkles, and tips of joints, muscles, and tendons will be observed with body movement, and can be used for locating points. For example:

- ST-6 Jiache is located one finger-width anterior and superior to the lower angle of the mandible and the prominence of the masseter muscle, when the teeth are clenched.

- SI-19 Tinggong is located between the tragus and the mandibular joint, where a depression is formed when the mouth is slightly open.

Finger measurement

The length and width of the patient's fingers are used as a criterion for locating points. The commonly used measuring methods are as follows:

- **Middle finger measurement:** When the middle finger is flexed, the distance between the two ends of the creases of the interphalangeal joints is taken as 1 cun (Figure 2.2), which is used to locate points on the four limbs and the back.

- **Thumb measurement:** The width of the interphalangeal joint of the thumb is taken as 1 cun (Figure 2.3), which is used to locate points on the four limbs and the back.

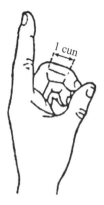

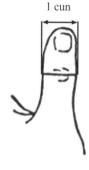

Figure 2.2 Middle finger measurement

Figure 2.3 Thumb measurement

- **Four fingers measurement:** The width of the four fingers (index, middle, ring, and little fingers), together, at the level of the skin crease of the proximal interphalangeal joint at the dorsum of the middle finger, is taken as 3 cun (Figure 2.4).

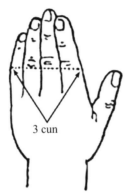

Figure 2.4 Four fingers measurement

EASY METHOD FOR LOCATING POINTS

The method for point location is easy to apply. For example, GB-31 Fengshi is located at the place that the tip of the middle finger touches, when the patient is standing erect with the hands close to the sides.

Points on the head

DU-20 BAIHUI

Location: On the vertex, 5 cun above the anterior hairline, on the midpoint of the line connecting the apexes of the two auricles (Figure 2.5). Patients should be in a sitting or lying position.

Indications: Headache, dizziness, hypertension, and prolapse of rectum.

Regional anatomy:

- Under the skin are subcutaneous tissue, galea aponeurotica, and loose tissue under galea aponeurotica.

- *Vasculature*: The anastomotic network formed by the superficial temporal arteries and veins and the occipital arteries and veins of both sides.

- *Innervation*: The branch of the great occipital nerve.

EX-HN-1 SISHENCONG

Location: A group of 4 points on the vertex, 1 cun respectively posterior, anterior and lateral to DU-20 Baihui (Figure 2.5).

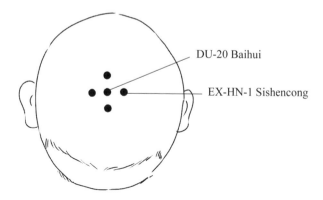

Figure 2.5

Indications: Headache, dizziness, insomnia, poor memory, and epilepsy.

Regional anatomy:

- Under the skin are subcutaneous tissue, galea aponeurotica, and loose tissue under galea aponeurotica.

- *Vasculature*: Occipital artery and vein, the parietal branch of the superficial temporal artery and vein, anastomosis of the supraorbital artery and vein.

- *Innervation*: Branches of the greater occipital nerve, auriculotemporal nerve and supraorbital nerve.

DU-17 NAOHU

Location: 2.5 cun superior to the posterior hairline, 1 cun above DU-16 Fengfu, superior to the external occipital protuberance (Figure 2.6).

Indications: Headache, dizziness, and optic neuritis.

Regional anatomy:

- Under the skin are subcutaneous tissue, the space between the two bellies of the occipitofrontal is muscle and loose tissue under galea aponeurotica.

- *Vasculature*: Branches of the occipital arteries and veins on both sides.

- *Innervation*: A branch of the great occipital nerve.

DU-21 QIANDING

Location: 3.5 cun within the anterior hairline, 1.5 cun anterior to DU-20 Baihui (Figure 2.6).

Indications: Headache, dizziness, epilepsy, swollen and inflamed face.

Regional anatomy:

- Under the skin are subcutaneous tissue, galea aponeurotica, and loose tissue under galea aponeurotica.

- *Vasculature*: Branches of the occipital arteries and veins on both sides.

- *Innervation*: A branch of the great occipital nerve.

DU-23 SHANGXING

Location: On the midline on the front of the head, 1 cun within the anterior hairline (Figure 2.6).

Indications: Headache, rhinitis, rhinorrhea, ophthalmalgia.

Regional anatomy:

- Under the skin are subcutaneous tissue, galea aponeurotica, and loose tissue under galea aponeurotica.

- *Vasculature*: Branches of the frontal artery and vein, branches of the superficial temporal artery and vein.

- *Innervation*: A branch of the frontal nerve.

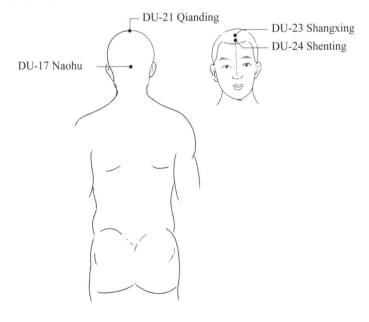

Figure 2.6

DU-24 SHENTING

Location: On the midline of the head, 0.5 cun within the anterior hairline (Figure 2.6).

Indications: Headache, dizziness, insomnia, rhinitis, epilepsy, and palpitation.

Regional anatomy:

- Under the skin are subcutaneous tissue, the occipito-frontal is muscle and loose tissue under galea aponeurotica.
- *Vasculature*: Branches of the frontal artery and vein.
- *Innervation*: A branch of the frontal nerve.

ST-8 TOUWEI

Location: On the lateral side of the head, 0.5 cun within the anterior hairline at the corner of the forehead, 4.5 cun lateral to the midline of the head (Figure 2.7).

Indications: Headache, blurred vision, dizziness, ophthalmalgia, and lacrimation.

Regional anatomy:

- Under the skin are subcutaneous tissue, galea aponeurotica inferior to the temporalis muscle, loose tissue under galea aponeurotica, and the periosteum of the skull.
- *Vasculature*: Frontal branches of the superficial temporal artery and vein.
- *Innervation*: A branch of the auriculotemporal nerve and the temporal branch of the facial nerve.

GB-3 SHANGGUAN

Location: In front of the ear, on the upper border of the zygomatic arch, in the depression directly above ST-7 Xiaguan (Figure 2.7).

Indications: Migraine, upper jaw toothache, and facial paralysis.

Regional anatomy:

- Under the skin are subcutaneous tissue, superficial and deep temporal fascia, and related loose tissue.
- *Vasculature*: Zygomatico-orbital artery and vein.
- *Innervation*: Zygomatico-orbital branch of the facial nerve and the zygomatico-facial nerve.

GB-4 HANYAN

Location: Within the hairline of the temporal region, midway of the upper half of the distance between ST-8 Touwei and GB-7 Qubin (Figure 2.7).

Indications: Migraine, tinnitus, dizziness, rhinitis, toothache, epilepsy, facial paralysis.

Regional anatomy:

- Under the skin are subcutaneous tissue, the auricularis superior muscle, temporal fascia, and the temporal muscle.

- *Vasculature*: The parietal branches of superficial temporal artery and vein.

- *Innervation*: The temporal branch of the auriculotemporal nerve.

GB-5 XUANLU

Location: Within the hairline of the temporal region, at the midpoint of the arc connecting ST-8 Touwei and GB-7 Qubin (Figure 2.7).

Indications: Migraine, facial edema, toothache, and neurasthenia.

Regional anatomy:

- Under the skin are subcutaneous tissue, the auricularis superior muscle, temporal fascia, and the temporalis muscle.

- *Vasculature*: The parietal branches of the superficial temporal artery and vein.

- *Innervation*: The temporal branch of the auriculotemporal nerve.

GB-6 XUANLI

Location: Within the hairline, inferior to the corner of the temporal region, midway between ST-8 Touwei and GB-7 Qubin (Figure 2.7).

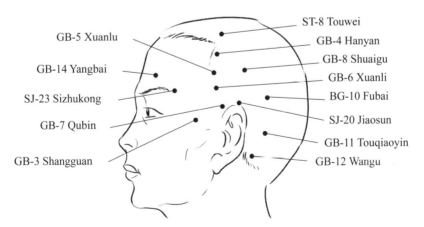

Figure 2.7

Indications: Migraine, facial edema, pain in the outer canthus, tinnitus, and upper-jaw toothache.

Regional anatomy:

- Under the skin are subcutaneous tissue, the auricularis superior muscle, temporal fascia, and the temporal muscle.

- *Vasculature*: The parietal branches of the superficial temporal artery and vein.

- *Innervation*: The temporal branch of the auriculotemporal nerve.

GB-7 QUBIN

Location: Within the hairline anterior and superior to the auricle, about one finger-width anterior to SJ-20 Jiaosun (Figure 2.7).

Indications: Headache, toothache, lockjaw, and sudden loss of voice.

Regional anatomy:

- Under the skin are subcutaneous tissue, the auricularis superior muscle, temporal fascia, and the temporalis muscle.

- *Vasculature*: The parietal branches of the superficial temporal artery and vein.

- *Innervation*: The temporal branch of the auriculotemporal nerve.

GB-8 SHUAIGU

Location: Superior to the apex of the auricle, 1.5 cun within the hairline (Figure 2.7).

Indications: Migraine, dizziness, infantile convulsions.

Regional anatomy:

- Under the skin are subcutaneous tissue, the auricularis superior muscle, temporal fascia, and the temporalis muscle.

- *Vasculature*: The parietal branches of the superficial temporal artery and vein.

- *Innervation*: The anastomotic branch of the auriculotemporal nerve and the great occipital nerve.

GB-10 FUBAI

Location: Posterior and superior to the mastoid process, in the middle of the curve line drawn from GB-9 Tianchong to GB-11 Touqiaoyin (Figure 2.7).

Indications: Headache, neck rigidity, tinnitus, toothache.

Regional anatomy:

- Under the skin are subcutaneous tissue and galea aponeurotica.
- *Vasculature*: The posterior auricular artery and vein.
- *Innervation*: The branch of the great occipital nerve.

GB-11 TOUQIAOYIN

Location: Posterior and superior to the mastoid process, on the line connecting GB-10 Fubai and GB-12 Wangu (Figure 2.7).

Indications: Headache, tinnitus, deafness, neck rigidity, and thyroid cysts.

Regional anatomy:

- Under the skin are subcutaneous tissue and galea aponeurotica.
- *Vasculature*: Branches of the posterior auricular artery and vein.
- *Innervation*: The anastomotic branch of the great and lesser occipital nerves.

GB-12 WANGU

Location: In the depression posterior and inferior to the mastoid process (Figure 2.7).

Indications: Headache, neck rigidity, swelling of the cheek, laryngalgia, facial paralysis, and parotitis.

Regional anatomy:

- Under the skin are subcutaneous tissue, the sternocleidomastoid muscle, splenius capitis muscle, and longissimus muscle.
- *Vasculature*: The posterior auricular artery and vein.
- *Innervation*: The lesser occipital nerve.

GB-13 BENSHEN

Location: 0.5 cun within the hairline of the forehead, at the junction of the medial two thirds and lateral one third of the distance from DU-24 Shenting to ST-8 Touwei (Figure 2.8).

Indications: Headache, blurred vision, and epilepsy.

Regional anatomy:

- Under the skin are subcutaneous tissue, galea aponeurotica, and the frontal belly of the occipito-frontal is muscle.
- *Vasculature*: Frontal braches of the superficial temporal artery and vein, the lateral branches of the frontal artery and vein.

- *Innervation*: The lateral branch of the frontal nerve.

GB-14 YANGBAI

Location: On the forehead, 1 cun above the midpoint of the eyebrow, approximately at the junction of the upper two-thirds and lower one third of the vertical line drawn from the anterior hairline to the eyebrow (Figure 2.7).

Indications: Headache, facial paralysis, and ophthalmopathy.

Regional anatomy:

- Under the skin are subcutaneous tissue and the frontal belly of the occipito-frontal is muscle.

- *Vasculature*: Lateral branches of the frontal artery and vein.

- *Innervation*: On the lateral branch of the frontal nerve.

GB-15 TOULINQI

Location: On the head, directly above the pupil, 0.5 cun within the anterior hairline, and 2.25 cun lateral the midline, midway between DU-24 Shenting and ST-8 Touwei (Figure 2.8).

Indications: Headache, lacrimation, blurred vision, nasal obstruction, and infantile convulsions.

Regional anatomy:

- Under the skin are subcutaneous tissue, galea aponeurotica, and loose tissue under galea aponeurotica.

- *Vasculature*: The frontal artery and vein.

- *Innervation*: The anastomotic branch of the medial and lateral branches of the frontal nerve.

SJ-20 JIAOSUN

Location: Directly above the ear apex, within the hairline of the temple (Figure 2.7).

Indications: Migraine, tinnitus, redness, swelling and pain of the eye, swelling of the cheek.

Regional anatomy:

- Under the skin are subcutaneous tissue, the auricularis superior muscle, temporal fascia, and the temporalis muscle.

- *Vasculature*: Branches of the superficial temporal artery and vein.

- *Innervation*: Branches of the auriculotemporal nerve.

SJ-23 SIZHUKONG

Location: In the depression at the lateral end of the eyebrow (Figure 2.7).

Indications: Headache, blurred vision, twitching of the eyelids, redness and pain in the eyes, toothache, and epilepsy.

Regional anatomy:

- Under the skin are subcutaneous tissue and the orbicularis muscle.
- *Vasculature*: Frontal branches of superficial temporal artery and vein.
- *Innervation*: The zygomatic branch of the facial nerve and a branch of the oculotemporal nerve.

BL-2 CUANZHU

Location: On the forehead, on the medial extremity of the eyebrow (Figure 2.8).

Indications: Headache, blurred vision, myopia, ptosis, facial paralysis.

Regional anatomy:

- Under the skin are subcutaneous tissue and orbicularis muscle.
- *Vasculature*: The frontal artery and vein.
- *Innervation*: The medial branch of the frontal nerve.

EX-HN-3 YINTANG

Location: Midway between the medial ends of the two eyebrows (Figure 2.8), when the patient is in the supine position.

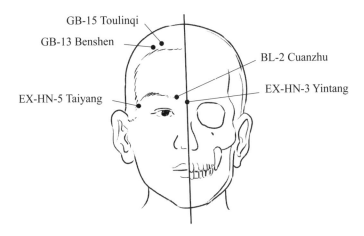

Figure 2.8

Indications: Infantile convulsions, headache, dizziness, rhinitis, rhinorrhea, and redness of the eyes.

Regional anatomy:

- Under the skin are subcutaneous tissue and the procerus muscle.
- *Vasculature*: A branch of the ophthalmic artery, frontal artery, and vein.
- *Innervation*: A branch of the frontal nerve and the supratrochlear nerve.

EX-HN-5 TAIYANG

Location: In the depression about 1 cun posterior to the midpoint between the lateral end of the eyebrow and the outer canthus (Figure 2.8).

Indications: Headache, migraine, facial paralysis, and ophthalmopathy.

Regional anatomy:

- Under the skin are subcutaneous tissue, the orbicularis muscle, temporal fascia, and temporalis muscle.
- *Vasculature*: Branches of the superficial temporal artery and vein.
- *Innervation*: Branch of the zygomatic nerve, temporal branch and zygomatic branch of the facial nerve, branch of the mandibular nerve.

Points on the neck and nape

GB-20 FENGCHI

Location: In the posterior aspect of the neck, below the occipital bone, in the depression between the upper portion of sternocleidomastoid and trapezius (Figure 2.9).

Indications: Headache, common cold, dizziness, stiffness and pain in the neck, red and painful eyes, and hypertension.

Regional anatomy:

- Under the skin are subcutaneous tissue, the space between sternocleidomastoid and trapezius, splenius capitis, semispinalis capitis, and the space between rectus capitis and obliquus capitis superior.
- *Vasculature*: Branches of the occipital artery and vein.
- *Innervation*: A branch of the lesser occipital nerve.

DU-15 YAMEN

Location: At the midpoint of the nape, in the depression 0.5 cun within the posterior hairline (Figure 2.9).

Indications: Epilepsy, sudden hoarseness of voice, stiffness of neck, and opisthotonus.

Regional anatomy:

- Under the skin are subcutaneous tissue, the space between the two sides of trapezius of the nuchal ligament, the space between the rectus capitis posterior major and minor muscles to either side.

- *Vasculature*: A branch of the occipital artery and vein, and the external vertebral venous plexus.

- *Innervation*: Branches of the third occipital nerve and the great occipital nerve, branches of the second and third posterior cervical nerves.

DU-16 FENGFU

Location: Directly below the external occipital protuberance, in the depression between the two sides of trapezius (Figure 2.9).

Indications: Headache, dizziness, neck rigidity, mental disorder, and sore throat.

Regional anatomy:

- Under the skin are subcutaneous tissue, tendons of both sides of trapezius of the nuchal ligament, the space between rectus capitis posterior major and minor to either side.

- *Vasculature*: A branch of the occipital artery.

- *Innervation*: Branches of the third occipital nerve and the great occipital nerve.

BL-10 TIANZHU

Location: On the nape, 1.3 cun lateral to the midline of the nape, within the posterior hairline, on the lateral side of trapezius (Figure 2.9).

Indications: Headache, stiffness of the nape, pain in the shoulder and back, mental disorder.

Regional anatomy:

- Under the skin are subcutaneous tissue, trapzius, splenius capitis, semispinalis capitis muscles.

- *Vasculature*: The occipital artery and vein.

- *Innervation*: The medial branch of the posterior branch of the third cervical nerve and the great occipital nerve.

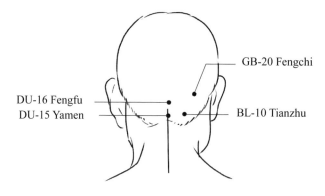

GB-20 Fengchi

DU-16 Fengfu
DU-15 Yamen

BL-10 Tianzhu

Figure 2.9

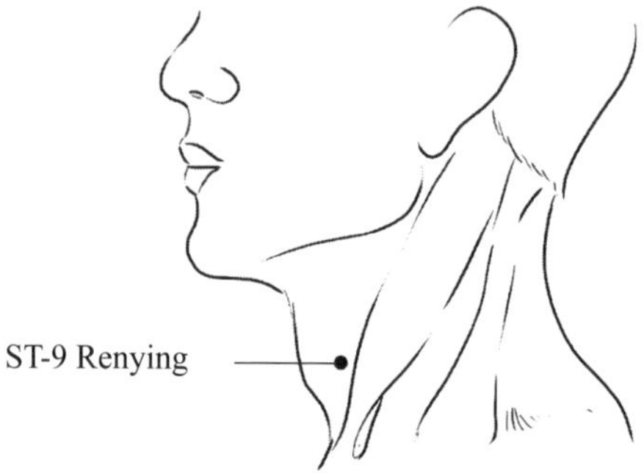

ST-9 Renying

Figure 2.10

ST-9 RENYING

Location: On the neck, level with the tip of the of Adam's apple, just on the course of the common carotid artery, on the anterior border of sternocleidomastoid (Figure 2.10).

Indications: Soreness and swelling of the throat, hypertension, headache, asthma, hemiparalysis, and scrofula.

Regional anatomy:

- Under the skin is subcutaneous tissue, the anterior border of sternocleidomastoid, and the posterior border of constrictor naris.

- *Vasculature*: The superior thyroid artery, the anterior jugular vein; laterally, the internal jugular vein; on the bifurcation of the internal and the external carotid arteries.

- *Innervation*: Superficially, the cutaneous cervical nerve, the cervical branch of the facial nerve; deeper, the sympathetic trunk; laterally, the descending branch of the hypoglossal nerve and the vagus nerve.

DU-14 DAZHUI

Location: Under the spinous process of the seventh cervical vertebra, approximately at the level of the shoulder (Figure 2.11).

Indications: Febrile diseases, malaria, sunstroke, stiffness of the neck and back, mental disorder.

Regional anatomy:

- Under the skin are subcutaneous tissue, the supraspinous ligaments, and the interspinous ligament.

- *Vasculature*: A branch of the transverse cervical artery.

- *Innervation*: The posterior ramus of the eighth cervical nerve and the medial branch of the posterior ramus of the first thoracic nerve.

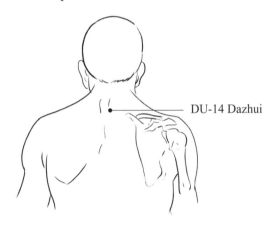

Figure 2.11

Points on the chest and abdomen

RN-4 GUANYUAN

Location: On the midline of the abdomen, 3 cun below the umbilicus (Figure 2.12).

Indications: Abdominal pain, leucorrhea, urinary tract infection, menstrual disorder, sexual dysfunction, health preservation (essence point for health preservation).

Regional anatomy:

- Under the skin are subcutaneous tissue, linea alba, transverse fascia, membrane of abdominal wall.

- *Vasculature*: Branches of the superficial epigastric and inferior epigastric arteries and veins.

- *Innervation*: The anterior branch and the anterior cutaneous branch of the 12th thoracic nerve.

RN-6 QIHAI

Location: On the midline of the abdomen, 1.5 cun below the umbilicus (Figure 2.12).

Indications: Abdominal distension, abdominal pain, diarrhea, and fatigue.

Regional anatomy:

- Under the skin are subcutaneous tissue, linea alba, transverse fascia, membrane of abdominal wall.

- *Vasculature*: Branches of the superficial epigastric and inferior epigastric arteries and veins.

- *Innervation*: The anterior cutaneous branch of the eleventh intercostal nerve.

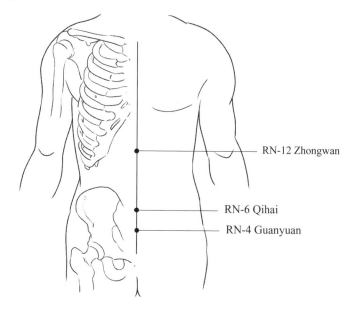

Figure 2.12

RN-12 ZHONGWAN

Location: On the midline of the abdomen, 4 cun above the umbilicus (Figure 2.12).

Indications: Gastric pain, chronic gastritis, gastric ulcer, gastroptosis, vomiting, hiccups, and schizophrenia.

REGIONAL ANATOMY:

- Under the skin are subcutaneous tissue, linea alba, transverse fascia, membrane of abdominal wall.
- *Vasculature*: The superior epigastric artery and vein.
- *Innervation*: The anterior cutaneous branch of the seventh intercostal nerve.

Points on the back

BL-15 XINSHU

Location: 1.5 cun lateral to the lower border of the spinous process of the fifth thoracic vertebra (Figure 2.13).

Indications: Insomnia, intercostal neuralgia, coronary heart disease, palpitations, mental disorder, and back pain.

Regional anatomy:

- Under the skin are subcutaneous tissue, and the trapezius, erector spinae, and sub-rhomboideus muscles.
- *Vasculature*: The medial cutaneous branches of the posterior branches of the intercostal artery and vein.
- *Innervation*: The medial cutaneous branches of the posterior rami of the fifth and sixth thoracic nerves; their lateral branches.

BL-17 GESHU

Location: 1.5 cun lateral to the lower border of the spinous process of the seventh thoracic vertebra (Figure 2.13).

Indications: Anemia, hemoptysis, vomiting, hiccup, asthma, and night sweating.

Regional anatomy:

- Under the skin are subcutaneous tissue, and the trapezius, erector spinae, and latissimus dorsi muscles.

- *Vasculature*: The medial cutaneous branches of the posterior branches of the intercostal artery and vein.

- *Innervation*: The medial cutaneous branches of the posterior rami of the seventh and eighth thoracic nerves, their lateral branches.

BL-18 GANSHU

Location: 1.5 cun lateral to the lower border of the spinous process of the ninth thoracic vertebra (Figure 2.13).

Indications: Jaundice, acute and chronic hepatitis, cholecystitis, ophthalmopathy, intercostal neuralgia, neurasthenia, depression, climacteric syndrome, menstrual disorder, and lower back pain.

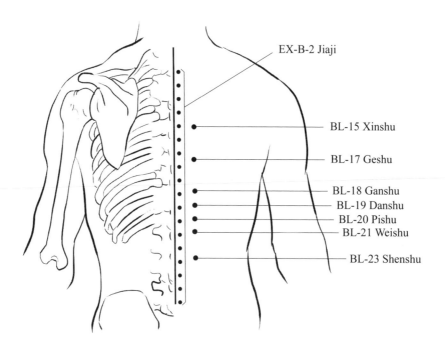

Figure 2.13

Regional anatomy:

- Under the skin are subcutaneous tissue, and the trapezius, latissimus dorsi, serratus posterior inferior, and erector spinae muscles.

- *Vasculature*: The medial branches of the posterior branches of the intercostal artery and vein.

- *Innervation*: The medial cutaneous branches of the posterior rami of the ninth and tenth thoracic nerves, their lateral branches.

BL-19 DANSHU

Location: 1.5 cun lateral to the lower border of the spinous process of the tenth thoracic vertebra (Figure 2.13).

Indications: Jaundice, bitter taste, pain in the hypochondriac region, and cholecystalgia.

Regional anatomy:

- Under the skin are subcutaneous tissue, and the trapezius, latissimus dorsi, serratus posterior inferior, and erector spinae muscles.

- *Vasculature*: The medial branches of the posterior branches of the intercostal artery and vein.

- *Innervation*: The medial cutaneous branches of the posterior rami of the tenth and eleventh thoracic nerves, their lateral branches.

BL-20 PISHU

Location: 1.5 cun lateral to the lower border of the spinous process of the eleventh thoracic vertebra (Figure 2.13).

Indications: Gastric disease, dyspepsia, neurogenic vomiting, enteritis, anemia, chronic hemorrhagic disease, and lower back pain.

Regional anatomy:

- Under the skin are subcutaneous tissue and the latissimus dorsi, serratus posterior inferior, and erector spinae muscles.

- *Vasculature*: The medial branches of the posterior branches of the intercostal artery and vein.

- *Innervation*: The medial cutaneous branches of the posterior rami of the eleventh and twelfth thoracic nerves, their lateral branches.

BL-21 WEISHU

Location: 1.5 cun lateral to the lower border of the spinous process of the twelfth thoracic vertebra (Figure 2.13).

Indications: Gastric pain, nausea, vomiting, abdominal distension, chest pain, and hypochondriac pain.

Regional anatomy:

- Under the skin are subcutaneous tissue, thoracolumbar fascia, fascia of latissimus dorsi and erector spinae muscles.

- *Vasculature*: The medial branches of the posterior branches of the subcostal artery and vein.

- *Innervation*: The medial cutaneous branches of the posterior rami of the twelfth thoracic nerve and first lumbar nerve, their lateral branches.

BL-23 SHENSHU

Location: 1.5 cun lateral to the lower border of the spinous process of the second lumbar vertebra (Figure 2.13).

Indications: Seminal emission, enuresis, menstrual disorder, asthma, tinnitus, deafness, hair loss, and lower back pain.

Regional anatomy:

- Under the skin are subcutaneous tissue, thoracolumbar fascia, fascia of latissimus dorsi and erector spinae muscles.

- *Vasculature*: The posterior rami of the second lumbar artery and vein.

- *Innervation*: The lateral cutaneous branch of the posterior ramus of the second and third lumbar nerves; deeper, its lateral branch.

EX-B-2 JIAJI

Location: A group of points on both sides of the spinal column at the lateral borders of each spinous process, from the first thoracic vertebra to the fifth lumbar vertebra (17 points), 0.5 cun lateral to midline of the back (Figure 2.13).

Indications: Lower back pain, dysfunction of Zang-Fu organs.

Regional anatomy:

- *Superficial layer*: Trapezius, latissimus dorsi, rhomboideus muscles.

- *Middle layer*: Serratus dorsalis, serratus ventralis muscles.

- *Deep layer*: Erector spinae and transversospinalis.

- *Vasculature and innervation*: The corresponding posterior rami of spinal nerves and their accompanying arteries and veins.

Points on the upper limbs

LI-4 HEGU

Location: Between the first and second metacarpal bones, approximately in the middle of the second metacarpal bone on the radial side (Figure 2.14).

Indications: Headache, red and swollen eyes, toothache, sore throat, rhinorrhagia, facial paralysis, deafness, parotitis, febrile disease, hidrosis, abdominal pain, constipation, amenorrhea, prolonged labor, numbness of upper limbs, urticant eruptions, and infantile convulsions.

Regional anatomy:

- Under the skin are subcutaneous tissue, the first dorsal interosseous muscle and the adductor hallucis muscle.

- *Vasculature*: The venous network of the dorsum of the hand; proximal to the point where the radial artery passes through the dorsum to the palm of the hand.

- *Innervation*: The superficial ramus of the radial nerve; deeper, the palmar digital proprial nerve derived from the median nerve.

LI-5 YANGXI

Location: On the radial side of the wrist. When the thumb is tilted upwards, it is in the depression between the tendons of extensor pollicis longus and brevis (Figure 2.14).

Indications: Headache, red and swollen eyes, toothache, sore throat, deafness, tinnitus, pain in the wrist, mania, and epilepsy.

Regional anatomy:

- Under the skin are subcutaneous tissue, and the tendon of extensor carpi radialis longus.

- *Vasculature*: The cephalic vein, the radial artery and its dorsal carpal branch.

- *Innervation*: The superficial ramus of the radial nerve.

LI-7 WENLIU

Location: With the elbow flexed, the point is 5 cun above transverse crease of wrist, on the line connecting LI-5 Yangxi and LI-11 Quchi (Figure 2.14).

Indications: Headache, facial swelling, sore throat, rhinorrhgia, shoulder and back pain, abdominal pain, mania, and pain in the upper limb.

Regional anatomy:

- Under the skin are subcutaneous tissue, antebrachial fascia, extensor carpi radialis longus and brevis.

- *Vasculature*: Muscular branch of the radial artery; the cephalic vein.

- *Innervation*: The posterior antebrachial cutaneous nerve and the deep ramus of the radial nerve.

LU-7 LIEQUE

Location: Superior to the styloid process of the radius, 1.5 cun above the transverse crease of the wrist (Figure 2.15).

Indications: Chronic pharyngitis, sore throat, common cold, asthma, rigidity of the neck, and facial paralysis.

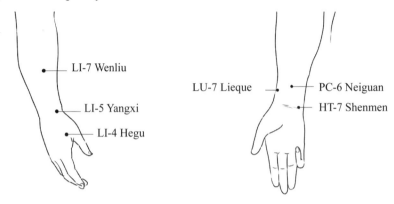

Figure 2.14   Figure 2.15

Regional anatomy:

- Under the skin are subcutaneous tissue, abductor pollicis longus, pronator quadratus and the radius.

- *Vasculature*: The cephalic vein, branches of the radial artery and vein.

- *Innervation*: The lateral antebrachial cutaneous nerve and the superficial ramus of the radial nerve.

HT-7 SHENMEN

Location: On the transverse crease of the wrist, in the articular region between the pisiform bone and the ulna, in the depression on the radial side of the tendon of flexor carpi ulnaris (Figure 2.15).

Indications: Cardiac pain, irritability, insomnia, poor memory, palpitation, dementia, mania, epilepsy, hypochondriac pain, yellowish sclera, feverish sensation in the palm, hematemesis, headache, dizziness and aphonia.

Regional anatomy:

- Under the skin are subcutaneous tissue, and tendon of flexor carpi ulnaris.

- *Vasculature*: The ulnar artery.

- *Innervation*: The medial antebrachial cutaneous nerve; on the ulnar side, the ulnar nerve.

PC-6 NEIGUAN

Location: 2 cun above the transverse crease of the wrist, between the tendons of palmaris longus and flexor carpi radialis (Figure 2.15).

Indications: Cardiac disease, mental disorder, gastric pain, vomiting, dizziness, and car sickness.

Regional anatomy:

- Under the skin are subcutaneous tissue, the space between the tendons of palmaris longus and flexor carpi radialis, flexor digitorum superficialis, flexor digitorum profundus, pronator quadratus, and the interosseous membrane of the forearm.

- *Vasculature*: The median artery and vein; deeper, the anterior interosseous artery and vein.

- *Innervation*: The medial and lateral antebranchial cutaneous nerves, the palmar cutaneous branch of the median nerve; deepest, the anterior interosseous nerve.

ST-11 QUCHI

Location: When the elbow is flexed, the point is in the depression at the lateral end of the transverse cubital crease (Figure 2.16).

Indications: Pain of the elbow and arm, motor impairment of the upper extremities, hypertension, fever, allergic disease, and dermatitis.

Regional anatomy:

- Under the skin are subcutaneous tissue, extensor carpi radialis longus and brevis, and brachioradialis.

- *Vasculature*: Branches of the radial recurrent artery and vein.

- *Innervation*: The posterior antebrachial cutaneous nerve; deeper on the medial side, the radial nerve.

SJ-5 WAIGUAN

Location: 2 cun above the transverse crease of the dorsal wrist, on the line connecting SJ-4 Yangchi and the olecranon, between the ulna and radius (Figure 2.17).

Indications: Febrile disease, deafness, tinnitus, headache, red and swelling pain, pain in the upper limb and the hypochondriac region.

Regional anatomy:

- Under the skin are subcutaneous tissue, extensor digiti minimi, extensor pollicis longus, and extensor indicis proprius.

- *Vasculature*: Deeper, the posterior and anterior interosseous arteries and veins.

- *Innervation*: The posterior antebrachial cutaneous nerve; deeper, the posterior interosseous nerve of the radial nerve, and the anterior interosseous nerve of the median nerve.

SJ-6 ZHIGOU

Location: 3 cun above the transverse crease of the dorsal wrist, on the line connecting SJ-4 Yangchi and the olecranon, between the ulna and radius (Figure 2.17).

Indications: Deafness, tinnitus, constipation, hypochondriac pain, and febrile disease.

Regional anatomy:

- Under the skin are subcutaneous tissue, extensor digiti minimi, extensor pollicis longus, and the interosseus membrane of the forearm.

- *Vasculature*: Deeper, the posterior and anterior interosseous arteries and veins.

- *Innervation*: The posterior antebrachial cutaneous nerve; deeper, the posterior interosseous nerve of the radial nerve, and the anterior interosseous nerve of the median nerve.

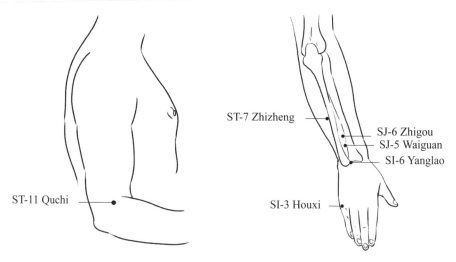

ST-7 Zhizheng

SJ-6 Zhigou
SJ-5 Waiguan
SI-6 Yanglao

ST-11 Quchi

SI-3 Houxi

Figure 2.16

Figure 2.17

SI-3 HOUXI

Location: When a loose fist is made, the point is proximal to the head of the fifth metacarpal bone on the ulnar side, in the depression at the junction of the red and white skin (Figure 2.17).

Indications: Headache, neck rigidity, contraction and twitching of elbow, arm and fingers, acute lumbar sprain, malaria, mania, and epilepsy.

Regional anatomy:

- Under the skin are subcutaneous tissue, abductor digiti minimi, and flexor brevis minimi digiti.

- *Vasculature*: The dorsal digital artery and vein, the dorsal venous network of the hand.

- *Innervation*: The dorsal branch derived from the ulnar nerve.

SI-6 YANGLAO

Location: Dorsal to the head of the ulna. On the radial side of the styloid process of the ulna (Figure 2.17).

Indications: Blurred vision and pain in the shoulder and upper limb.

Regional anatomy:

- Under the skin are subcutaneous tissue, the tendon of extensor carpi ulnaris.

- *Vasculature*: The terminal branches of the posterior interosseous artery and vein, the dorsal venous network of the wrist.

- *Innervation*: The anastomotic branches of the posterior antebrachial cutaneous nerve and the dorsal branch of the ulnar nerve.

SI-7 ZHIZHENG

Location: 5 cun proximal to the transverse crease of dorsal wrist, on the line connecting SI-5 Yanggu and SI-8 Xiaohai (Figure 2.17).

Indication: Neck stiffness, contracture and twitching of elbow, pain in finger, headache, febrile disease, blurrd vision, poor memory, and excessive thirst.

Regional anatomy:

- Under the skin are subcutaneous tissue, flexor carpi ulnaris, flexor digitorum profundus, and the interosseus membrane of the forcarm.

- *Vasculature*: The terminal branch of the posterior interosseous artery and vein.

- *Innervation*: Superficially, the branch of the medial antebrachial cutaneous nerve; deeper, on the radial side, the posterior interosseous nerve.

Points on the lower limbs

ST-36 ZUSANLI

Location: 3 cun below ST-35 Dubi, one finger-width from the anterior crest of the tibia (Figure 2.18).

Indications: Gastric pain, vomiting, nausea, acute/chronic gastroenteritis, numbness in the lower limbs, arthritis, hypertension, etc.

Regional anatomy:

- Under the skin are subcutaneous tissue, tibialis anteriora, the interosseous membrane of the leg, and tibialis posterior.
- *Vasculature*: The anterior tibial artery and vein.
- *Innervation*: Superficially, the lateral sural cutaneous nerve and the cutaneous branch of the saphenous nerve; deeper, the deep peroneal nerve.

ST-37 SHANGJUXU

Location: 6 cun below ST-35 Dubi, one finger-width from the anterior crest of the tibia (Figure 2.18).

Indications: Abdominal pain, diarrhea, constipation, appendicitis, pain and numbness in the lower limbs.

Regional anatomy:

- Under the skin are subcutaneous tissue, tibialis anterior, interosseous membrane of the leg, and tibialis posterior.
- *Vasculature*: The anterior tibial artery and vein.
- *Innervation*: Superficially, the lateral sural cutaneous nerve and the cutaneous branch of the saphenous nerve; deeper, the deep peroneal nerve.

ST-39 XIAJUXU

Location: 9 cun below ST-35 Dubi, about one finger-width from the anterior crest of the tibia (Figure 2.18).

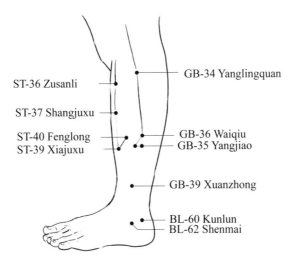

Figure 2.18

Indications: Lower abdominal pain, diarrhea, dysentery, pain and paralysis of the lower extremities.

Regional anatomy:

*   Under the skin are subcutaneous tissue, tibialis anterior, interosseous membrane of the leg, and tibialis posterior.

*   *Vasculature*: The anterior tibial artery and vein.

*   *Innervation*: Branches of the superficial peroneal nerve and the deep peroneal nerve.

ST-40 FENGLONG

Location: 8 cun superior and anterior to the external malleolus, about two finger-widths from the anterior crest of the tibia (Figure 2.18).

Indications: Excessive sputum, headache, dizziness, hypertension, vomiting, constipation, mental disorder, pain and paralysis of the lower extremities.

Regional anatomy:

*   Under the skin are subcutaneous tissue, extensor digitorum longus, interosseous membrane of the leg, and tibialis posterior.

*   *Vasculature*: The branches of the anterior tibial artery and vein.

*   *Innervation*: The superficial peroneal nerve.

ST-44 NEITING

Location: On the dorsum of the foot, proximal to the web margin between the second and third toes (Figure 2.19).

Indications: Toothache, nasal bleeding, laryngalgia, abdominal distension, viral dysentery, and nettle rash.

Regional anatomy:

- Under the skin are subcutaneous tissue, between the second and third tendons of extensor digitorum longus.
- *Vasculature*: The dorsal venous network of the foot.
- *Innervation*: The lateral branch of the medial dorsal cutaneous nerve divides into the dorsal digital nerves.

ST-45 LIDUI

Location: On the lateral side of the second toe, about 0.1 cun posterior to the corner of the nail (Figure 2.19).

Indications: Mental disorder, dream-disturbed sleep, febrile diseases, facial swelling, deviation of the mouth, and toothache.

Regional anatomy:

- Under the skin are subcutaneous tissue and the nail root.
- *Vasculature*: The arterial and venous network formed by the dorsal digital artery and vein of the foot.
- *Innervation*: The dorsal digital nerve derived from the superficial peroneal nerve.

GB-34 YANGLINGQUAN

Location: In the depression anterior and inferior to the head of the fibula (Figure 2.18).

Indications: Hepatobiliary diseases, hypertension, numbness and pain of the lower extremities, and hemiplegia.

Regional anatomy:

- Under the skin are subcutaneous tissue, peroneus longus, and extensor digitorum longus.
- *Vasculature*: The inferior lateral genicular artery and vein.
- *Innervation*: The common peroneal nerve bifurcates into the superficial and deep peroneal nerves.

GB-35 YANGJIAO

Location: 7 cun above the tip of the external malleolus, on the posterior border of the fibula (Figure 2.18).

Indications: Knee pain, muscular atrophy, pleurisy, and hepatitis.

Regional anatomy:

- Under the skin are subcutaneous tissue, gastrocnemius, and peroneus longus.

- *Vasculature*: The branches of the peroneal artery and vein.

- *Innervation*: The lateral sural cutaneous nerve.

GB-36 WAIQIU

Location: 7 cun above the tip of the external malleolus, on the anterior border of the fibula (Figure 2.18).

Indications: Pain in the leg, chest, and hypochondriac region.

Regional anatomy:

- Under the skin are subcutaneous tissue, peroneus longus and brevis, extensor digitorum longus, and peroneus longus.

- *Vasculature*: Branches of the anterior tibial artery and vein.

- *Innervation*: The superficial peroneal nerve.

GB-39 XUANZHONG

Location: 3 cun above the tip of the external malleolus, in the depression between the posterior border of the fibula and the tendons of peroneus longus and brevis (Figure 2.18).

Indications: Hemiplegia, lumbar and back pain, menstrual disorder, and hypertension.

Regional anatomy:

- Under the skin are subcutaneous tissue, extensor digitorum longus, and the interosseous membrane.

- *Vasculature*: Branches of the anterior tibial artery and vein.

- *Innervation*: The superficial peroneal nerve.

GB-40 QIUXU

Location: Anterior and inferior to the external malleolus, in the depression on the lateral side of the tendon of extensor digitorum longus (Figure 2.19).

Indications: Pain and swelling in the ankle joint, hemiplegia, and cholecystis.

Regional anatomy:

- Under the skin are subcutaneous tissue, extensor brevis digitorum, the lateral talo-calcaneal ligament, and tarsal sinus.

- *Vasculature*: A branch of the anterolateral malleolar artery.

- *Innervation*: Branches of the intermediate dorsal cutaneous nerve and superficial peroneal nerve.

GB-41 ZULINQI

Location: In the depression distal to the junction of the fourth and fifth metatarsal bones, on the lateral side of the tendon of extensor digiti minimi of the foot (Figure 2.19).

Indications: Headache, eye pain, distending pain of the breast, and pain in the costal and hypochondriac region.

Regional anatomy:

- Under the skin are subcutaneous tissue, fourth dorsal interossei, and third plantar interossei.

- *Vasculature*: The dorsal arterial and venous network of the foot, the fourth dorsal metatarsal artery and vein.

- *Innervation*: A branch of the intermediate dorsal cutaneous nerve of the foot.

GB-43 XIAXI

Location: Between the fourth and fifth toes, proximal to the margin of the web (Figure 2.19).

Indications: Headache, tinnitus, dizziness, hypertension, pain in the costal and hypochondriac region, and hemiplegia.

Regional anatomy:

- Under the skin are subcutaneous tissue, fourth tendon of extensor digitorum longus/brevis, and fifth tendon of extensor digitorum longus/brevis.

- *Vasculature*: The dorsal digital artery and vein.

- *Innervation*: The dorsal digital nerve.

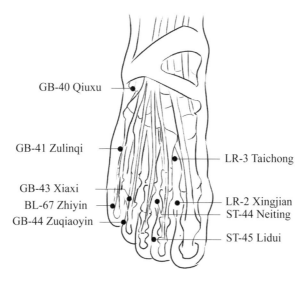

GB-40 Qiuxu

GB-41 Zulinqi

LR-3 Taichong

GB-43 Xiaxi
BL-67 Zhiyin
GB-44 Zuqiaoyin

LR-2 Xingjian
ST-44 Neiting

ST-45 Lidui

Figure 2.19

GB-44 ZUQIAOYIN

Location: On the lateral side of the fourth toe, about 0.1 cun posterior to the corner of the nail (Figure 2.19).

Indications: Migraine, ophthalmalgia, febrile disease, hypertension, and pain in the hypochondriac region.

Regional anatomy:

- Under the skin are subcutaneous tissue and the nail root.

- *Vasculature*: The arterial and venous network formed by the dorsal digital artery and vein and plantar digital artery and vein.

- *Innervation*: The dorsal digital nerve.

BL-60 KUNLUN

Location: In the depression between the tip of the external malleolus and Achilles tendon (Figure 2.18).

Indications: Headache, neck rigidity, back pain, and pain in the heel.

Regional anatomy:

- Under the skin are subcutaneous tissue and loose connective tissue.

- *Vasculature*: The external malleolar arterial network.

- *Innervation*: The sural nerve.

BL-62 SHENMAI

Location: In the depression directly below the external malleolus (Figure 2.18).

Indications: Epilepsy, mental disorder, headache, dizziness, insomnia, back pain, swelling and pain of the lower extremities.

Regional anatomy:

- Under the skin are subcutaneous tissue, tendon of peroneus longus and brevis, lateral talo-calcaneal ligament.

- *Vasculature*: The external malleolar arterial network, saphenous vein.

- *Innervation*: The sural nerve and cutaneous dorsalis lateralis nerve.

BL-67 ZHIYIN

Location: On the lateral side of the small toe, about 0.1 cun posterior to the corner of the nail (Figure 2.19).

Indications: Headache, nasal obstruction, malaria, ophthalmagia, difficult labour, and fetal malposition.

Regional anatomy:

- Under the skin are subcutaneous tissue and the nail root.

- *Vasculature*: The network formed by the dorsal digital artery and plantar digital proprial artery.

- *Innervation*: The plantar digital proprial nerve and the lateral dorsal cutaneous nerve of the foot.

LR-2 XINGJIAN

Location: Between the first and second toe, proximal to the margin of the web (Figure 2.19).

Indications: Headache, blurred vision, red and swollen eyes, menorrhagia, urethralgia, retention of urine, deviation of mouth, epilepsy, convulsions and dysmenorrhea, leukorrhea, and wind stroke.

Regional anatomy:

- Under the skin are subcutaneous tissue, the basilar part of the proximal phalanx of the hallux (big toe) and the head of second metatarsal bone.

- *Vasculature*: The dorsal venous network of the foot and the first dorsal digital artery and vein.

- *Innervation*: The site where the dorsal digital nerves split from the deep peroneal nerve.

LR-3 TAICHONG

Location: In the depression distal to the junction of the first and second metatarsal bones (Figure 2.19).

Indications: Headache, dizziness, red and swollen eyes, menstrual disorder, functional urine bleeding, infantile convulsions, hernia, epilepsy, and numbness of lower limb.

Regional anatomy:

- Under the skin are subcutaneous tissue, tendon of extensor digitorum longus, extensor hallucis longus, and first dorsal interossei.

- *Vasculature*: The dorsal venous network of the foot, the first dorsal metatarsal artery.

- *Innervation*: Branch of the deep peroneal nerve.

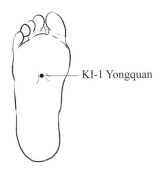

Figure 2.20

KI-1 YONGQUAN

Location: In the depression appearing on the sole when the foot is in plantar flexion, approximately at the junction of the anterior and middle third of the sole (Figure 2.20).

Indications: Coma, syncope, mania, infantile convulsions, headache, insomnia, incontinence of urine, and constipation.

Regional anatomy:

- Under the skin are subcutaneous tissue, the plantar aponeurosis, and the second lumbrical muscle.

- *Vasculature*: Deeper, the plantar arch.

- *Innervation*: The second common plantar digital nerve.

KI-3 TAIXI

Location: In the depression between the medial malleolus and tendo calcaneus, level with the tip of the medial malleolus (Figure 2.22).

Indications: Headache, blurred vision, deafness, toochache, insomnia, poor memory, sexual disorder, nocturia, and lower back pain with leg pain.

Regional anatomy:

- Under the skin are subcutaneous tissue, tendons of tibialis posterior, flexor digitorum longus, and calcaneus, the plantaris tendon, and flexor hallucis longus.

- *Vasculature*: Anteriorly, the posterior tibial artery and vein.

- *Innervation*: The medial crural cutaneous nerve, on the course of the tibial nerve.

KI-7 FULIU

Location: 2 cun directly above KI-3 Taixi, on the anterior border of tendo calcaneus (Figure 2.22).

Indications: Edema, night sweating, febrile disease, abdominal distension, diarrhea, pain in the lower limbs, and hemiplegia.

Regional anatomy:

- Under the skin are subcutaneous tissue, the tendon of tibialis posterior, the tendon of flexor digitorum longus, tendo calcaneus, the plantaris tendon, and extensor hallucis longus.

- *Vasculature*: Deeper, anteriorly, the posterior tibial artery and vein.

- *Innervation*: The medial sural and medial crural cutaneous nerves; deeper, the tibial nerve.

SP-3 TAIBAI

Location: On the medial side of the foot, proximal and inferior to the head of the first metatarsal bone, at the junction of the red and white skin (Figure 2.21).

Indications: Abdominal distension, gastric pain, diarrhea, and joint pain.

Regional anatomy:

- Under the skin are subcutaneous tissue, abductor hallucis, and flexor hallucis brevis.

- *Vasculature*: The dorsal venous network of the foot, the medial plantar artery, and branches of the medial tarsal artery.

- *Innervation*: Branches of the saphenous nerve and superficial peroneal nerve.

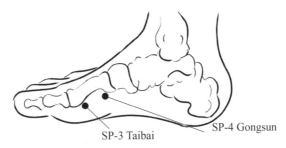

SP-4 Gongsun

SP-3 Taibai

Figure 2.21

SP-4 GONGSUN

Location: In the depression distal and inferior to the base of the first metatarsal bone, at the junction of the red and white skin (Figure 2.21).

Indications: Gastric pain, vomiting, abdominal distension, and diarrhea.

Regional anatomy:

- Under the skin are subcutaneous tissue, abductor hallucis, flexor hallucis brevis, and the flexor longus muscle tendon.

- *Vasculature*: The medial tarsal artery and the dorsal venous network of the foot.

- *Innervation*: The saphenous nerve and a branch of the superficial peroneal nerve.

SP-6 SANYINJIAO

Location: 3 cun directly above the tip of the medial malleolus, on the posterior border of the tibia, on the line between the medial malleolus and SP-9 Yinlingquan (Figure 2.22).

Indications: Abdominal distension, diarrhea, dysmenorrhea, menstrual disorder, leucorrhea, sexual disorder, enuresis, insomnia, hypertension, and dermatosis.

Regional anatomy:

- Under the skin are subcutaneous tissue, flexor digitorum longus, tibialis posterior, and extensor hallucis longus.

- *Vasculature*: The great saphenous vein, the posterior tibial artery and vein.

- *Innervation*: Superficially, the medial crural cutaneous nerve; deeper, in the posterior aspect, the tibial nerve.

SP-9 YINLINGQUAN

Location: On the lower border of the medial condyle of the tibia, in the depression between the posterior border of the tibia and gastrocnemius (Figure 2.22).

Indications: Edema, abdominal distension, diarrhea, jaundice, urinary incontinence, and pain in the knee joint.

Regional anatomy:

- Under the skin are subcutaneous tissue, semimembranosus, semitendinosus, and the medial head of gastrocnemius.

- *Vasculature*: Anteriorly, the great saphenous vein, the genu suprema artery; deeper, the posterior tibial artery and vein.

- *Innervation*: Superficially, the medial crural cutaneous nerve; deeper, the tibial nerve.

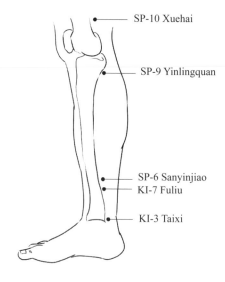

Figure 2.22

SP-10 XUEHAI

Location: On the medial side of the leg, 2 cun above the medio-superior border of the patella, on the bulge of the medial portion of quadriceps femoris, when the knee is flexed (Figure 2.22).

Indications: Menstrual disorder, metrorrhegia, functional uterine bleeding, amenorrhea, eczema, and urticaria.

Regional anatomy:

- Under the skin are subcutaneous tissue and vastus medialis.

- *Vasculature*: The muscular branches of the femoral artery and vein.

- *Innervation*: The anterior femoral cutaneous nerve and the muscular branch of the femoral nerve.

Chapter *3*

Acupuncture Therapies for Treating Migraine

Migraine is recommended for treatment using acupuncture by the World Health Organization (WHO). It achieves obvious therapeutic benefits with few side effects. Therefore, acupuncture is already an important therapy in the treatment of migraine.

Section I Common Acupuncture Methods

Migraine is classified into the patterns outlined below, according to the patient's clinical symptoms.

Filiform needle therapy

Filiform needle therapy is shown in Figure 3.1.

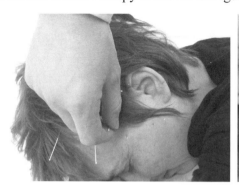 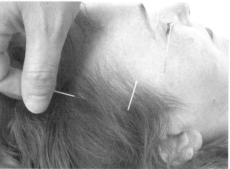

Figure 3.1 Filiform needle therapy

VISCERAL SYNDROME DIFFERENTIATION

Headache due to liver yang

Main symptoms: Pain and distension in the head, vexation, agitation, red eyes, bitter taste in the mouth.

Accompanying symptoms: Red face, dry mouth, red tongue with yellow coating, wiry or wiry rapid pulse.

Treatment principles: Calm the liver, extinguish wind to free the collateral vessels and reduce pain.

Acupoints: GB-20 Fengchi, SJ-20 Jiaosun, LR-2 Xingjian, GB-44 Zuqiaoyin, GB-8 Shuaigu (Figure 3.2).

Notes: In the treatment of headache due to liver yang:

- GB-20 Fengchi is used to harmonize qi and blood, regulate meridians and collaterals, expel wind, clear heat, and open orifices.

- SJ-20 Jiaosun is used to clear the head, improve vision, expel wind, and activate collaterals.

- LR-2 Xingjian and GB-44 Zuqiaoyin are used to clear heat, reduce fire, and regulate meridians.

- GB-8 Shuaigu is used to activate blood circulation and it is a key acupoint in treating migraine.

All acupoints are combined to clear heat, reduce fire, calm the liver, and extinguish wind.

Manipulation: Disinfect the skin of the area to be treated in the normal way. Insert the needle perpendicularly to a depth of 1.5 cun, and manipulate the needle according to reinforcing or reducing methods when the qi arrives.

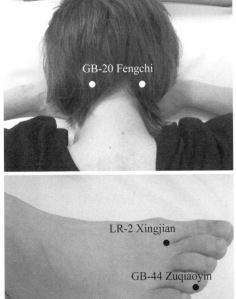
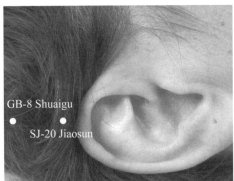

Figure 3.2 Acupoints for headache due to liver yang

Duration of treatment: Needles are retained for 30 minutes. The treatment is given once a day, and ten times forms a course of treatment.

Headache due to kidney deficiency

Main symptoms: Empty pain in the head, dizziness, lower back pain, weak knees, vexing heat in the five hearts (two hands, two feet, and heart).

Accompanying symptoms: Lassitude, lack of strength, tinnitus, red tongue with reduced coating, deep, thready, and weak pulse.

Treatment principles: Nourish kidney yin, tonify qi, and relieve pain.

Acupoints: DU-20 Baihui, DU-4 Mingmen, RN-4 Guanyuan, ST-36 Zusanli (Figure 3.3).

Notes:

- DU-20 Baihui is used to restore yang, to stop collapse, and benefit the brain, and tranquilize.

- DU-4 Mingmen is used to nourish the kidney and benefit yang.

- RN-4 Guanyuan, which is the source of Sanjiao, is used to nourish the kidney qi.
- ST-36 Zusanli, Sea point of the Stomach Meridian, is a key point for maintaining postnatal health.

All points combine to nourish the kidney essence and warm yang.

Manipulation: Disinfect the skin of the area to be treated in the normal way. Insert the needle perpendicularly to a depth of 1.5 cun, and manipulate the needle according to reinforcing or reducing methods when the qi arrives.

Duration of treatment: Needles are retained for 30 minutes. The treatment is given once a day, and ten times forms a course of treatment.

Headache due to qi deficiency

Main symptoms: Recurrent dull pain in the head, symptoms becoming severe due to tiredness.

Accompanying symptoms: Palpitations, poor appetite, spontaneous sweating, shortness of breath, lassitude, lack of strength, pale complexion, pale tongue with thin, white coating, deep, thready, and weak pulse.

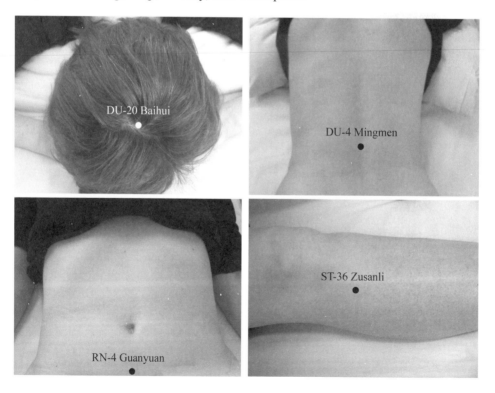

Figure 3.3 Acupoints for headache due to kidney deficiency

Treatment principles: Nourish qi and blood to relieve pain.

Acupoints: RN-6 Qihai, BL-20 Pishu, DU-20 Baihui, RN-8 Shenque, ST-36 Zusanli (Figure 3.4).

Notes:

- BL-20 Pishu, Back-Shu point of the spleen, is the postnatal source of the body. It is used to strengthen the spleen and benefit transformation.

- DU-20 Baihui, the meeting point of all the yang, is used to lift the yang qi of the entire body to assist its transportation and transformation.

- RN-8 Shenque is used to harmonize the stomach and the spleen, as well as to warm yang.

- RN-6 Qihai and ST-36 Zusanli are points to strengthen the body.

All points are used to generate qi and blood, improve general physical condition, and relieve headache.

Manipulation: Disinfect the skin of the area to be treated in the normal way. Insert the needle perpendicularly to a depth of 1.5 cun and manipulate the needle according to reinforcing or reducing methods when the qi arrives.

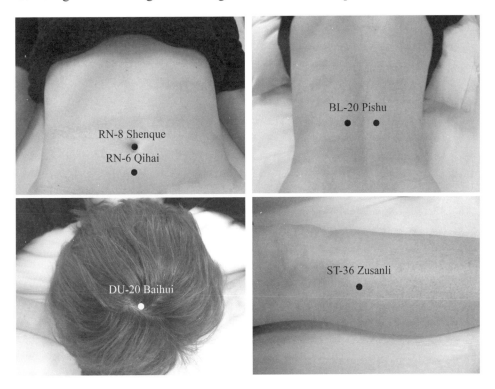

Figure 3.4 Acupoints for headache due to qi deficiency

Duration of treatment: Needles are retained for 30 minutes. The treatment is given once a day, and ten times forms a course of treatment.

Headache due to blood stasis

Main symptoms: Persistent stabbing pain and fixed pain.

Accompanying symptoms: Dark purple or spotty tongue; thin, white tongue coating; deep, thready or choppy, thready pulse.

Treatment principles: Activate the blood and resolve stasis, dredge channels, and relieve pain.

Acupoints: GB-20 Fengchi, LR-3 Taichong, BL-17 Geshu, EX-HN-3 Yintang, EX-HN-1 Sishencong, Ashi points (Figure 3.5).

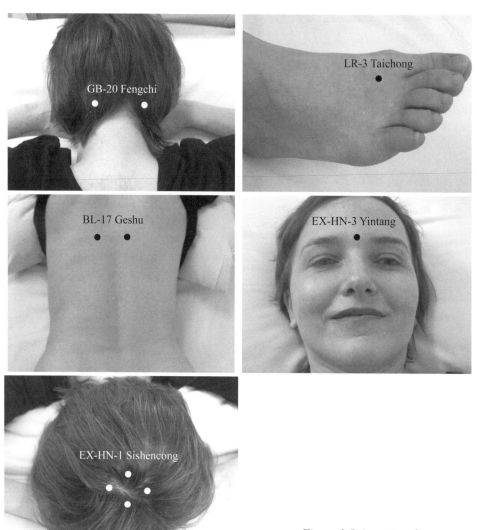

*Figure 3.5 Acupoints for
headache due to blood stasis*

Notes:

- Ashi points, EX-HN-3 Yintang, and EX-HN-1 Sishencong are used to activate meridian qi locally.

- GB-20 Fengchi is used to open orifices, dredge channels, and activate collaterals.

- LR-3 Taichong is used to soothe the liver and regulate qi and blood circulation, to resolve stasis.

- BL-17 Geshu, the meeting point of the blood, is good at activating the blood and resolving stasis.

All acupoints combine to resolve blood stasis and relieve headache.

Manipulation: Disinfect the skin of the area to be treated in the normal way. Insert the needle perpendicularly to a depth of 1.5 cun and manipulate the needle according to reinforcing or reducing methods when the qi arrives.

Duration of treatment: Needles are retained for 30 minutes. The treatment is given once a day, and ten times forms a course of treatment.

Headache due to phlegm turbidity

Main symptoms: Heavy sensation in the head, oppression in the chest and abdomen, nausea, and vomiting with phlegm.

Accompanying symptoms: Bland taste in the mouth, poor appetite, enlarged tongue with white, greasy coating, wiry, slippery pulse.

Treatment principles: To dry dampness and resolve phlegm, dredge channels, and relieve pain.

Acupoints: ST-8 Touwei, EX-HN-5 Taiyang, ST-40 Fenglong, RN-12 Zhongwan, ST-36 Zusanli, SP-9 Yinlingquan (Figure 3.6).

Notes:

- ST-8 Touwei and EX-HN-5 Taiyang are selected as the key points in treating migraine. Both acupoints are used to regulate stagnated meridian qi locally.

- ST-40 Fenglong, RN-12 Zhongwan, ST-36 Zusanli, and SP-9 Yinlingquan are used to invigorate spleen and harmonize stomach, bring qi down, and resolve phlegm.

- The combination of RN-12 Zhongwan and ST-36 Zusanli, is considered as a key acupoint combination to resolve phlegm.

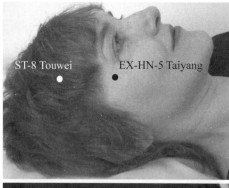
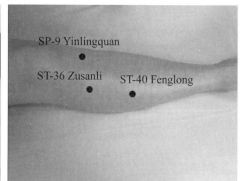
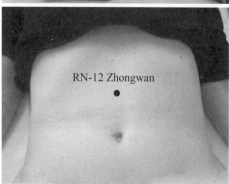

*Figure 3.6 Acupoints for headache
due to phlegm turbidity*

Manipulation: Disinfect the skin of the area to be treated in the normal way. Insert the needle perpendicularly to a depth of 1.5 cun and manipulate the needle according to reinforcing or reducing methods when the qi arrives.

Duration of treatment: Needles are retained for 30 minutes. The treatment is given once a day, and ten times forms a course of treatment.

MERIDIAN PATTERN DIFFERENTIATION

The human head is divided into different regions according to the meridian pathways (meridian pattern differentiation). The forehead and the supraorbital ridge belong to the Yangming Meridian. The back of the head belongs to the Taiyang Meridian. The apex of the head belongs to the Jueyin Meridian. The side of the head belongs to the Shaoyang Meridian.

It is clear that, as migraine pain is on the side of the head, it belongs to the Shaoyang Meridian. Pain in other parts of the head may also present in some cases. Therefore, the meridian pattern differentiation of migraine is related mainly to the Shaoyang Meridian, and may also be related to other meridians.

Shaoyang Meridian headache

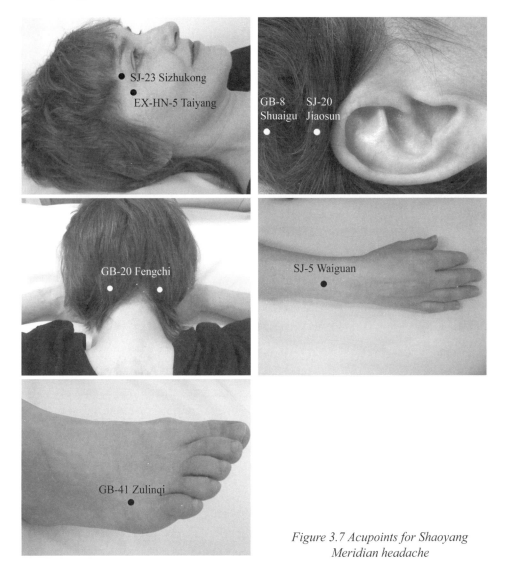

Figure 3.7 Acupoints for Shaoyang Meridian headache

Various clinical symptoms may present. The pain is usually on one or both sides of the head; it occurs on the side of the head for most patients. It is the pathway of the Shaoyang Sanjiao Meridian of the Hand and the Shaoyang Gallbladder Meridian of the Foot. The accompanying symptoms of the Shaoyang Gallbladder Meridian of the Foot include nausea, vomiting, bitter taste in the mouth, acid reflux, and increased saliva. Therefore, the pain region and symptoms show a close relationship with the Shaoyang Meridian, and so acupoints of the Shaoyang Meridian are selected as the main points for treating migraine.

Treatment principles: To disperse the Shaoyang Meridian, extinguish wind, and relieve pain.

Acupoints: EX-HN-5 Taiyang, SJ-23 Sizhukong, SJ-20 Jiaosun, GB-8 Shuaigu, GB-20 Fengchi, SJ-5 Waiguan, GB-41 Zulinqi (Figure 3.7).

Notes: EX-HN-5 Taiyang is an effective extra point in treating headache. The other acupoints belong to the Shaoyang Meridian. The treating principle is to regulate the Shaoyang Meridian.

Manipulation: Disinfect the skin of the area to be treated in the normal way. Insert the needle perpendicularly on EX-HN-5 Taiyang, GB-20 Fengchi, SJ-5 Waiguan, GB-41 Zulinqi. The needling angle on GB-20 Fengchi should be aimed towards the contralateral eye corner. Apply transverse needling on other acupoints. Manipulate the needle according to patient's condition: reducing methods are used for excessive cases, and reinforcing methods on deficient cases. Apply moxibustion when it is necessary. Neutral reinforcement and reduction is used for patients with no obvious excessive or deficient symptoms.

Duration of treatment: Needles are retained for 30 minutes. Manipulate the needle every ten minutes. The treatment is given once a day for acute headache, and every other day for chronic headache. Ten times forms a course of treatment.

Yangming Meridian headache

In most cases, the pain is in the forehead. Sometimes the pain also spreads to the occipital region, the apex of the head, the orbital region, or even radiates to the face, neck, or shoulder. Pain in the forehead and the orbital region belongs to Yangming Meridian headache.

Treatment principles: To clear and reduce the Yangming Meridian, relax the bowels, and relieve pain.

Acupoints: LI-4 Hegu, LI-5 Yangxi, LI-7 Wenliu, LI-8 Xialian, LI-9 Shanglian, ST-2 Sibai, ST-8 Touwei, ST-40 Fenglong, ST-41 Jiexi, ST-44 Neiting, RN-12 Zhongwan (Figure 3.8).

Notes: The acupoints selected in the treatment belong to the Yangming Meridian except for RN-12 Zhongwan. The aim is to dredge the Yangming Meridian. RN-12 Zhongwan of the Conception Channel is an alarm point of the stomach. It is the point where stomach qi is transported into the chest and the abdomen. Therefore, reducing methods are applied on RN-12 Zhongwan to clear stomach heat and to regulate qi and the blood of Yangming Meridian, in order to relieve pain in the forehead.

Manipulation: Disinfect the skin of the area to be treated in the normal way. Insert the needles perpendicularly and apply reducing methods on the needles.

Duration of treatment: Needles are retained for 30 minutes. Manipulate the needles every ten minutes. The treatment is given once a day for acute headache, and every other day for chronic headache. Ten times forms a course of treatment.

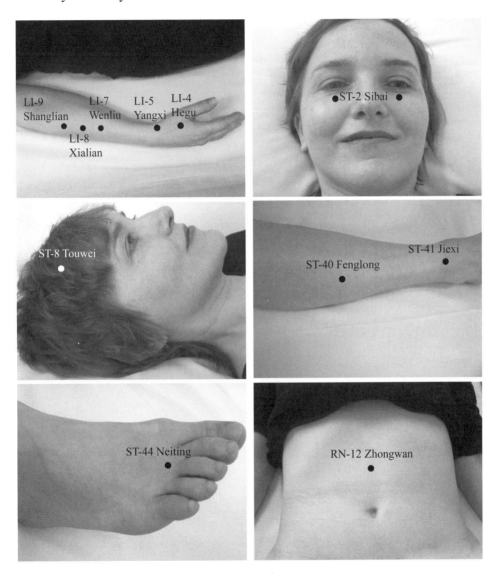

Figure 3.8 Acupoints for Yangming Meridian headache

Jueyin Meridian headache

Some patients suffer from pain on the apex of the head. This is caused by wind-cold invading the Liver Meridian. It is also caused by ascendant hyperactivity of liver yang. The Liver Meridian and the Governor Channel meet at the apex of the head. Coldness ascends along the meridian and disturbs clear yang, or causes hyperactivity of liver yang. Both of them inhibit circulation of qi and blood. Usually, agitated patients conform to this pattern

Treatment principles: To pacify the liver and extinguish wind, regulate meridians and collaterals.

Acupoints: LR-2 Xingjian, LR-3 Taichong, DU-20 Baihui, EX-HN-1 Sishencong, LI-4 Hegu (Figure 3.9).

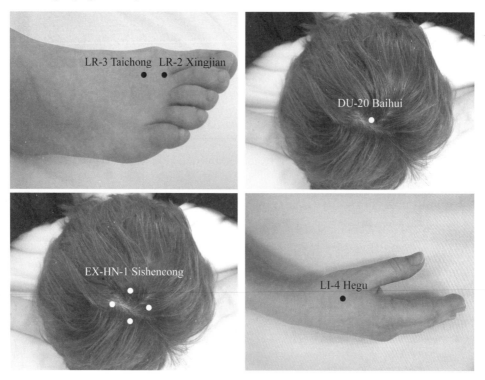

Figure 3.9 Acupoints for Jueyin Meridian headache

Notes:

- DU-20 Baihui and EX-HN-1 Sishencong are effective acupoints in treating pain on the apex of the head.

- LI-4 Hegu is used to harmonize the stomach and resolve dampness. LR-3 Taichong, source point of the Jueyin Liver Meridian, is used to soothe the liver qi.

- The combination of LI-4 Hegu and LR-3 Taichong is called "Four Gate Acupoints."

- Apply bloodletting therapy on EX-HN-1 Sishencong for ascendant hyperactivity of liver yang patients. It has instant effect and decreases blood pressure.

Manipulation: Disinfect the skin of the area to be treated in the normal way. Insert the needle perpendicularly on LR-2 Xingjian and LR-3 Taichong. Apply transverse needling on other acupoints. Manipulate the needles according to the patient's condition: reducing methods are used on excessive patients, and reinforcing methods on deficient patients. Apply moxibustion when necessary. Neutral reinforcement and reduction is used for patients with no obvious excessive or deficient symptoms.

Duration of treatment: Needles are retained for 30 minutes. Manipulate the needle every ten minutes. The treatment is once a day for acute headache, and every other day for chronic headache. Ten times forms a course of treatment.

Taiyang Meridian headache

Some patients suffer from pain on the back of the head. It is usually caused by wind cold invading the Taiyang Meridian. Common symptoms are headache attack with pain radiating to the neck and shoulder. It is accompanied by a series of wind cold symptoms.

Treatment principles: To disperse wind, dissipate cold, and regulate meridians.

Acupoints: SI-4 Wangu, SI-3 Houxi, SI-2 Qiangu, SI-7 Zhizheng, SI-8 Xiaohai, BL-2 Cuanzhu, BL-3 Meichong, BL-60 Kunlun, GB-20 Fengchi, DU-16 Fengfu (Figure 3.10).

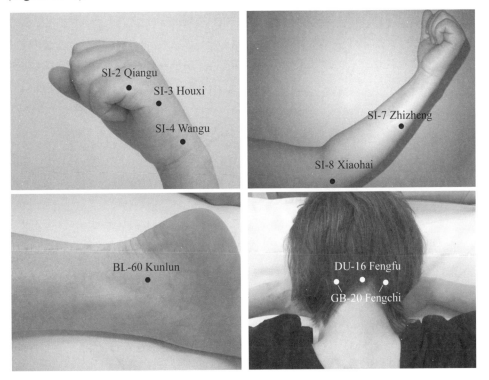

Figure 3.10 Acupoints for Taiyang Meridian headache

Notes: GB-20 Fengchi and DU-16 Fengfu are effective local acupoints. Other acupoints of the Taiyang Meridian are used to regulate the Taiyang Meridian.

Manipulation: Disinfect the skin of the area to be treated in the normal way. Insert the needle perpendicularly on acupoints, except for BL-2 Cuanzhu and BL-3 Meichong. Pay attention to the needling angle and the depth of GB-20 Fengchi and DU-16 Fengfu. Apply transverse needling on the other acupoints. Manipulate the needle according to patient's condition: reducing methods are used for excessive patients, and reinforcing methods on deficient patients. Apply moxibustion when necessary. Neutral reinforcement and reduction is used for patients with no obvious excessive or deficient symptoms.

Duration of treatment: Needles are retained for 30 minutes. Manipulate the needles every ten minutes. The treatment is given once a day for acute headache, and every other day for chronic headache. Ten times forms a course of treatment.

OTHER THERAPIES

Hua Tuo Jiaji points

Jiaji points, or Hua Tuo Jiaji points, are acupoints 0.5 cun lateral to the spinal process from vertebrae T1 to L5. These acupoints achieve an effect similar to that of the Back-Shu points. Their nerve regulation function is better than that of the Back-Shu points. The needle manipulation of Hua Tuo Jiaji points is safer than for Back-Shu points since these points are closer to the spine.

Using Hua Tuo Jiaji points in the treatment of migraine is based on visceral syndrome differentiation. Back-Shu points are selected, since they are effective in directly regulating the related Zang-Fu organs, instead of the traditional meridian pattern differentiation. Migraine is a disease that results from vegetative nerve dysfunction. Stimulating Hua Tuo Jiaji points is a good and safe way to regulate the nerve function.

Acupoints: GB-20 Fengchi, Hua Tuo Jiaji points (T5, 7, 9, 11, 14) (Figure 3.11).

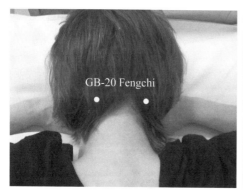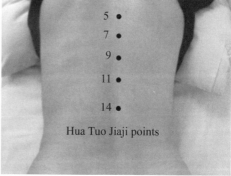

Figure 3.11 Hua Tuo Jiaji points

Notes: Hua Tuo Jiaji points (T5, 7, 9, 11, 14) are similar to BL-15 Xinshu, BL-17 Geshu, BL-18 Ganshu, BL-20 Pishu, and BL-23 Shenshu. The Zang-Fu organs are closely related to the onset of migraine. For example, "all (syndromes characterized by) pain, itching and sores are associated with the heart," and so migraine is related to the heart. BL-17 Geshu is the meeting point of blood. Migraine due to blood stasis is related to BL-17 Geshu. "Spleen deficiency generates phlegm," and so migraine due to phlegm turbidity is related to the spleen. Migraine due to liver and kidney deficiency is related to the liver and the kidney. Therefore, a safe method is to regulate Zang-Fu organ function in order to relieve headache. It is suitable for all types of migraine, especially for menstrual migraine.

Manipulation: Disinfect the skin of the area to be treated in the normal way. Insert a 1.5 cun needle on GB-20 Fengchi, with the needle tip aiming towards the contralateral eye corner, for about 1 cun transversely. Manipulate the needle when the qi arrives. Make the needling sensation spread to the forehead or the temple region of the same side of the head along the Shaoyang Meridian; then remove the needle. Ask the patient to lie in the prone position when puncturing Hua Tuo Jiaji points. Position the tip of the needle obliquely towards to the spine for about 1 cun. The needling sensation will be transmitted along the spine or the ribs.

Duration of treatment: Needles are retained for 30 minutes. The treatment is given once a day, and 30 times forms a course of treatment.

Starting and terminal points of meridians

Root-tip theory and branch-foundation theory are first recorded in the book of *Huangdi Neijing*: *Miraculous Pivot, Discussion on Root-tip Theory, and Discussion on Defensive Qi*. Starting and terminal points refer to qi gathering and spreading in 12 meridians. The branch-foundation theory considers the head, face, and trunk as the branch, and the four limbs as the foundation. The three "tips," or gatherings, lie on the head (for three yang meridians of the hand or foot), chest (for the three yin meridians of the hand) and abdomen (for the three yin meridians of the foot.). Overall, the root-tip and branch-foundation theories show the close relation between the four limbs and the head and trunk of the body. They emphasize that the four limbs are the source of meridian qi, and show the importance of acupoints on the four limbs, especially those below the elbow and the knee, in clinical practice.

Migraine pain is located on the head. It belongs to branch *and* tip, and so both the root and the foundation should be used in the treatment. Acupoints should be selected from below the elbow or the knee, and should also include acupoints on the head.

Acupoints: SJ-23 Sizhukong, GB-8 Shuaigu, SJ-19 Luxi, SJ-3 Zhongzhu, GB-41 Zulinqi, GB-44 Zuqiaoyin (Figure 3.12).

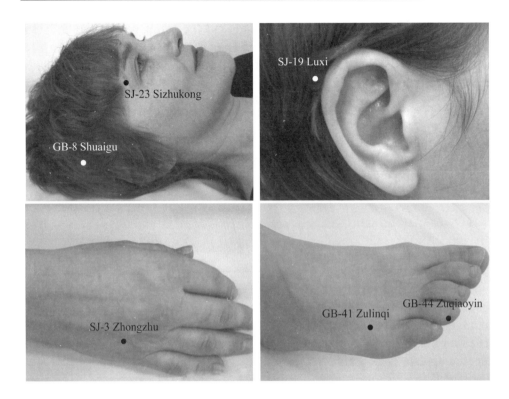

Figure 3.12 Starting and terminal points of meridians

Notes:

- If qi is in reverse motion, disease that is located in the upper part of the body can be cured by treating the lower part of the body; disease that is located in the lower part of the body can be cured by treating the upper part of the body; disease that is located in the middle of the body can be cured by treating the lateral side of the body (as set out in the book of *Huangdi Neijing: Plain Questions, Major Discussion on the Administration of Five-Motions*).

- Contralateral channel needling is used on SJ-3 Zhongzhu, GB-41 Zulinqi, and GB-44 Zuqiaoyin. SJ-3 Zhongzhu belongs to the Sanjiao Meridian. GB-41 Zulinqi and GB-44 Zuqiaoyin are the stream point and well point of the Gallbladder Meridian respectively. The three acupoints are located on the tip of the four limbs, which are the root or the foundation. These points are used to clear heat, pacify the liver, and extinguish wind.

- SJ-23 Sizhukong, GB-8 Shuaigu and SJ-19 Luxi are Gallbladder Meridian points on the head. They belong to tip and branch. These points are used to dredge meridians and relieve pain.

Acupoints from the upper part of the body and the lower part of the body are combined, in root-tip theory, to regulate the meridians of the entire body so as to harmonize qi and blood circulation and relieve pain. This approach is suitable for treating all types of migraine.

Manipulation: Ask the patient to take a sitting position. Disinfect the skin of the area to be treated in the normal way. Insert a 1 cun needle on SJ-23 Sizhukong, GB-8 Shuaigu, SJ-19 Luxi, to a depth of 2–3 fen. Twirl the needle with mild reinforcement and reduction. Contralateral channel needling is used on SJ-3 Zhongzhu, GB-41 Zulinqi and GB-44 Zuqiaoyin. Insert a 1 cun needle to a depth of 3–5 fen. Lift and thrust the needle with mild reinforcement and reduction.

Duration of treatment: Needles are retained for 15–20 minutes. Treatment is given once a day, and ten times forms a course of treatment.

Contralateral collateral needling

Contralateral collateral needling was first applied in the method of Miuci. It treats disease on the left side by needling the acupoints on the right side, and disease on the right side by needling the acupoints on the left side. If there is pain and the disease does not involve any channel, the method of Miuci is used. The acupuncturist must inspect the skin to see if there is blood stasis in the collaterals. If there is blood stasis in the collaterals, they are needled to let out blood. (The book of *Huangdi Neijing*: *Plain Questions, Discussion on Contralateral Needling Therapy* indicates that acupoint selection for contralateral collateral needling uses acupoints on the right to treat symptoms of the left side, and acupoints on the left side to treat problems on the right side: the disease is located on the contralateral collateral. It also shows that the indication for contralateral collateral needling is pain of the body with the absence of an apparent abnormal pulse, which means that the disease is limited to the collateral level.)

Most migraine presents with the symptom of pain on one side of the head and no obvious abnormal pulse. It is a disease of collateral and is suitable for contralateral collateral needling.

Acupoints:

- *Main points*: GB-8 Shuaigu, GB-20 Fengchi, EX-HN-5 Taiyang, Hegu (all points on the healthy side).

- *Combined points*: GB-34 Yanglingquan, LR-3 Taichong, SJ-5 Waiguan, GB-41 Zulinqi (all points on the healthy side) (Figure 3.13).

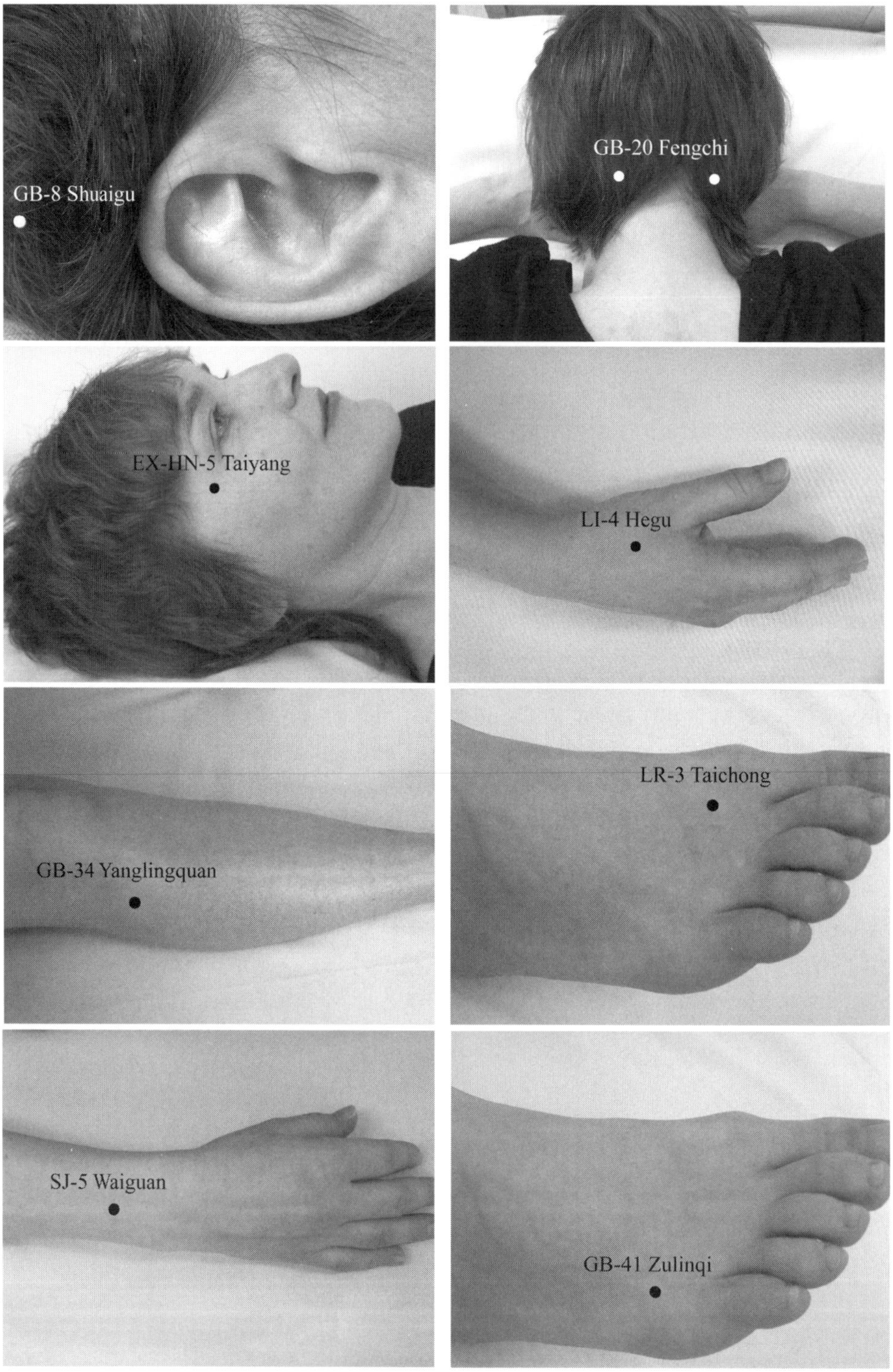

GB-8 Shuaigu

GB-20 Fengchi

EX-HN-5 Taiyang

LI-4 Hegu

GB-34 Yanglingquan

LR-3 Taichong

SJ-5 Waiguan

GB-41 Zulinqi

Figure 3.13 Contralateral collateral needling

Notes: Migraine is a disease that affects the Shaoyang Meridian. Therefore, the acupoint selection is mainly from the Shaoyang Meridian. However, the contralateral Shaoyang Meridian and acupoints are used in the treatment. This method is suitable for short-term migraine when there is no obvious abnormal pulse.

Manipulation: Apply routine needling method. Twirl the needle with strong stimulation for reducing when qi arrives.

Duration of treatment: Needles are retained for 30 minutes. Manipulate the needles every ten minutes. The treatment is given once a day, and ten times forms a course of treatment.

Bio-holographic therapy

Second metacarpal holographic therapy is a method of needling acupoints on the radial side of the second metacarpal bone to treat disease in the whole body. This method, which originated from bio-holographic theory, was founded by Professor Zhang Yingqing. Bio-holographic theory holds that an organism is formed by holographic parts in different developmental phases.

The second metacarpal holographic acupoints are points on the radial side of the second metacarpal bone between the head and the base of the bone. The 12 acupoints are head, neck, upper limbs, lung and heart, liver, stomach, duodenum, kidneys, lower back, lower abdomen, leg, and foot. The second metacarpal is a miniature of the human body. Each acupoint treats diseases related to its Zang-Fu organ.

The disease area of migraine is the head. Therefore, according to bio-holographic theory, point selection should be related to the head.

Acupoints: Use an acupoint of the hand on the same side as the headache: it is the shallow depression on the radial side, close to the head of the second metacarpal bone (Figure 3.14).

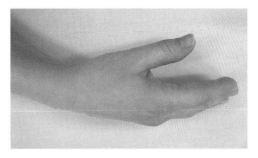

Figure 3.14 Bio-holographic therapy

Notes: Research shows that needling the bio-holographic points can raise one's pain threshold and pain tolerance. It is effective in relieving acute pain. The point targeting the head is selected. It is effective in treating all types of migraine.

Manipulation: Apply routine needling method. Insert a 1 cun needle to a depth of 0.5 cun. Lift and thrust or twirl the needle with neutral reinforcement and reduction.

Duration of treatment: Needles are retained for 30 minutes. Manipulate the needles every five minutes. The treatment is given once a day and ten times forms a course of treatment.

Ear acupuncture

Ear acupuncture uses filiform needles or other methods to stimulate the ear points to prevent and treat diseases (Figure 3.15 and 3.17). The ear is closely related to the three yang meridians of the hand and the three yang meridians of the foot. Although the six yin meridians do not directly enter into the ear, they connect with the ear via divergences which join the Yang Meridian – and so the 12 meridians are all directly or indirectly connected with the ear. The ear is closely related to the Zang-Fu organ. The shape and color changes of the ear also reveal diseases of the Zang-Fu organ and assist diagnosis and treatment.

EAR SEED APPLICATION

Ear seed application (Figure 3.15) is the mildest stimulation, and the most common of all ear therapies. The specific ear point is constantly stimulated by a Wangbuliuxing (*semen vaccariae*), which is fixed in place by a piece of sticking plaster. This method is well-accepted by patients because of the low risk of infection, less pain, and no injury of the skin.

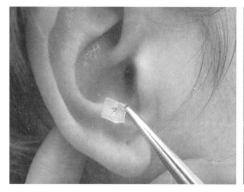 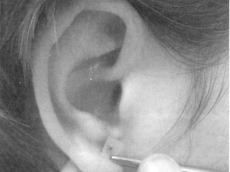

Figure 3.15 Ear seed application

Point selection should follow syndrome differentiation. Ear acupuncture theory is based on bio-holographic theory, and supported by several other theories.

Therefore, the point should be selected from the affected region (as well as following the guidance of both Chinese medicine and modern medicine). This type of point selection is accepted because it treats both the cause and the symptoms of a disease.

In point selection, some points target the symptom of migraine, and other points are used to treat the accompanying symptoms. The latter indicate the abnormal Zang-Fu organ (or the system and organ abnormality, in modern medicine). For example, copious sweating indicates heart and lung disorders. Insomnia and lots of dream activity indicate heart and kidney problems. Abundant phlegm and heavy limbs indicate spleen disorder. Combined points are selected to achieve better therapeutic results.

Acupoints: Shenmen, Subcortex, Liver, Gallbladder, Temple, Forehead, plus Heart and Kidney for dizziness, insomnia, and restlessness, and Stomach and Sympathetic for nausea and vomiting (Figure 3.16).

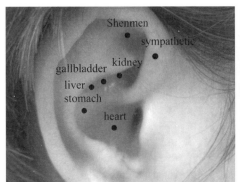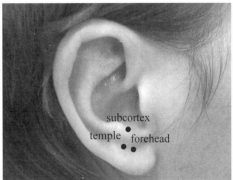

Figure 3.16 Acupoints for ear seed application

Notes: Shenmen is effective at tranquilizing and relieving pain. It is a key point in treating headache. Subcortex is used to regulate the nervous system. Forehead and Temple are used to benefit the brain. The effect will be enhanced when combined with Shenmen. Migraine is closely related to the liver and gallbladder in Chinese medicine (syndrome differentiation), so these are the main points in the treatment. Other points are combined, considering the symptoms and their related Zang-Fu organs. This method is effective in treating all types of migraine, since all symptoms are taken into account in this treatment plan.

Manipulation: This method searches for the tender spots on the ear with a probe. Disinfect the skin in the normal way. Lay Wangbuliuxing (*semen vaccariae*) on the point with a piece of plaster. Press the tender point to produce pain and a burning sensation on the auricle.

Duration of treatment: Keep the ear seed application in place for 3–5 days. Press the seed on the ear 5–10 times a day, and 5–10 minutes each time. Treat both ears alternately each week. Ten weeks form a course of treatment.

EAR NEEDLING

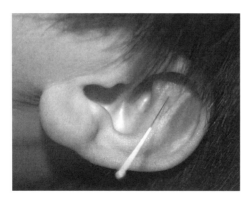

Figure 3.17 Ear needling

Ear needling (Figure 3.17) gives more stimulation than seed application, and also requires more technique. A unique feature of the auricle of the ear is that there is no muscle layer. The needle reaches cartilage directly after penetrating the skin. Any malpractice will easily cause infection, and recovery from infection is also difficult. Therefore, strict disinfection should be followed.

The needle should be inserted quickly, and the needling angle should be between 15 and 30 degrees. Mild stimulation requires transverse insertion, which only penetrates the skin. Strong stimulation requires the needle to pierce the cartilage, but without touching the skin below the cartilage.

Needling the ear is more directly effective and quicker than seed application, and gives effective, long-term pain relief.

Ear needling is usually used to treat severe migraine, and uses a number of acupoints.

Acupoints: Forehead, Temple, Occipital, Shenmen, Sympathetic or Subcortex, Liver or Gallbladder, Kidney or Stomach (Figure 3.18).

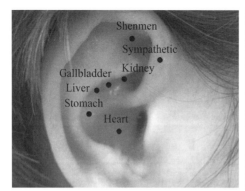
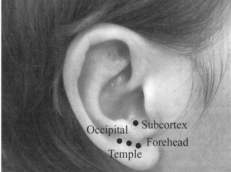

Figure 3.18

Notes: There is no obvious difference between needling and seed application for point location and syndrome differentiation. The needling technique penetrates to a deeper layer of the ear to give stronger stimulation. The pain-relieving effect is also stronger than with seed application. It is suitable for treating medium to severe attacks of migraine.

Manipulation: Search for tender points in the acupoint region to locate the acupoint. Disinfect the skin in the normal way. Hold the auricle with the left hand and insert the short filiform needle with the right hand. The needling depth should be within the cartilage but not right through it. Manipulate the needle with medium stimulation. Twirl the needle quickly when qi arrives.

Duration of treatment: Needles are retained for 30 minutes. Manipulate the needles twice during the treatment, five minutes each time. Treat both ears alternately every day. Twenty times form a treating course.

Bloodletting therapy

Bloodletting therapy has a long history. In the earliest records of three-edged needling, it is called "collateral needling," "repeated shallow needling," or "leopard-spot needling" (*Huangdi Neijing*: *Miraculous Pivot, Discussion on Official Needling Techniques*). The therapeutic mechanism of three-edged needling is recorded in the book of *Huangdi Neijing*: *Miraculous Pivot, Discussion on Filiform Needles*, which says that bloodletting therapy should be used to treat blood stasis (Figure 3.19).

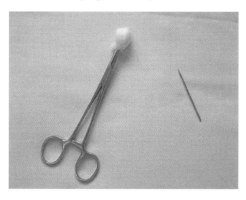

Figure 3.19 Bloodletting therapy

THE POINT-PRICKING METHOD

The point-pricking method is the technique of squeezing the skin around the acupoint to gather blood in the acupoint. Disinfect the acupoint and rapidly prick it for about 1–2 fen with the right hand. Then squeeze around the point to collect blood. The mild stimulation and slight bleeding activate meridian qi to promote qi and blood circulation. Clinical practice proves that bloodletting on the head or around the ear is an effective method for treating headache. This method gives instant pain relief for headache.

Acupoints: Ashi points, EX-HN-5 Taiyang, tender points of the Shaoyang Meridian (Figure 3.20).

Notes: Traditional Chinese Medicine holds that pain is caused by blockage. Search for tender points on the Shaoyang Meridian to find the blockage in the meridian. Pricking the point for blood reduces evil qi which is blocking the meridian, and regulates the Shaoyang Meridian. Pricking for blood on an Ashi point regulates the meridian on the head to relieve pain. Protect the needling hole from contact with water for 24 hours after bloodletting therapy, and clean the region around it to prevent infection. This method is suitable for excessive pattern migraine. Beware of using bloodletting therapy for hemophiliac patients, or patients with fear of blood.

Manipulation: Choose one or two Ashi points and two or three tender points of the Shaoyang Meridian for each treatment. (The number of points should not exceed four in each treatment.) Disinfect the skin in the normal way. Prick the acupoint with a three-edged needle or disposable injection needle. Squeeze out some blood (or combine with cupping for bleeding). Press the needling hole with a piece of dry cotton and sterilize the local region.

Duration of treatment: The treatment is given every other day, and ten times forms a course of treatment.

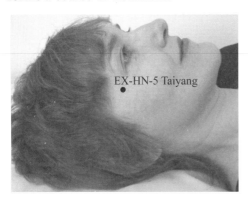

Figure 3.20 Acupoints for the point-pricking method

COLLATERAL BLOODLETTING

Collateral bloodletting, or collateral needling, is a method of puncturing a superficial vein for a small amount of blood, after disinfection. It is a common method in treating migraine. Obvious purple veins are presented around EX-HN-5 Taiyang or SJ-23 Sizhukong in most migraine patients. It is recorded in the book of *Acupuncture Collection of Mianxuetang* that in migraine cases obvious purple collaterals are presented on EX-HN-5 Taiyang, and that bloodletting therapy should be used in the treatment. The enlarged small veins are called "Taiyang purple veins" or "collaterals" in Chinese medicine. Pricking for blood in this area aims to dispel stasis to promote regeneration.

Acupoints: EX-HN-5 Taiyang, ST-8 Touwei, GB-4 Hanyan, GB-5 Xuanlu, GB-6 Xuanli, GB-7 Qubin, Ashi (all acupoints are selected on the affected side) (Figure 3.21).

Notes: Chinese medicine holds that chronic disease affects the blood and collaterals. Stasis should be removed by bloodletting. Modern research shows that needling collaterals regulates collaterals and harmonizes qi and blood. It also clears all types of pathogens that may harm the brain collateral. Collateral bloodletting treats the pain, as well as the cause of the headache. It is suitable for migraine due to excessive pattern and chronic deficiency-excess in complexity. It is effective in relieving pain during an attack. Avoid using bloodletting therapy for patients with abnormal coagulation, hemophilia, or fear of blood.

Manipulation: Select one or two acupoints to use each time. Search for the obvious vein on or around the acupoint, and tap it lightly for puncturing. Disinfect the acupoint and fix it with the left hand. Prick the vein rapidly with a three-edged needle (or disposable injection needle) for blood. Let the bleeding stop by itself. The bleeding amount should be 1–2ml. Squeeze the local area to increase bleeding if the blood is not enough.

Duration of treatment: The treatment is given once every three days, and seven times forms a course of treatment.

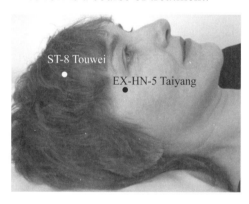

Figure 3.21 Acupoints for collateral bloodletting

THE PIERCING METHOD

The piercing method is a method of pressing or holding the disinfected skin with the left hand and pricking the acupoint or reflective points for blood or pus with a needle held in the right hand. Or insert the needle 0.5 fen deeper to break some of the fibers to treat the disease. The strong stimulation is effective in eliminating blood stasis and regulating meridians. It is suitable for severe headache.

Acupoints: Use the frontal and parietal branches of the superficial temporal artery on the affected side. Locate separate points on the two branches; the distance between the two points should be about the width of one finger. Tap the local area if the collaterals are not obvious (Figure 3.22).

Notes: This method is originated from the recording of the book of *Huangdi Neijing*: *Miraculous Pivot, Discussion on Meridians*. It is recorded that if puncturing the collaterals, the obvious blood vessels must be selected and punctured. The pricking is at the separation of blood vessels since they are the region where blood vessels accumulated, or called blood stasis in Chinese medicine. Clinical practice receives good therapeutic effect by using this method. It is suitable for long-term and severe migraine. The effect is good for blood stasis pattern migraine. Be careful when using bloodletting therapy for patients with abnormal coagulation, hemophilia, diabetes, fear of blood, or low pain tolerance.

Manipulation: Five to 15 points are used each time. More points (more than ten) can be used for first-time patients with a strong constitution and severe headache. Reduce the number of points for other patients (5–7 points). Disinfect the skin in the normal way and prick the skin with a three-edged needle (or disposable injection needle). The tip of the needle is at an angle of 20–30 degrees to the skin. The needle is first inserted into the skin for about 1.5mm. Prick the skin. Then prick the deeper fibers below the skin, as far as the blood vessel wall. Prick the blood vessel wall superficially for 1–2 drops of blood. Press to stop bleeding if it produces too much blood. Start pricking from the distal part when the collateral is obvious and beating. Prick from the near part towards the distal part when the collaterals are not obvious. Disinfect the point with iodine after pricking.

Duration of treatment: The treatment is given once every three days, and three times forms a course of treatment.

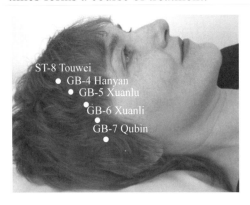

Figure 3.22 Acupoints for the piercing method

Moxibustion

Moxibustion is a therapeutic method of preventing and treating disease by burning moxa wool or herbal medicine on or over acupoints or the affected area of the body (Figure 3.23). The warm stimulation and the effect of medicinal herbs regulate qi and blood circulation and expel evil factors. Moxibustion is an external therapy for diseases for which acupuncture is not effective. Moxibustion warms the meridian, especially on the head, to relieve pain.

The use of moxibustion in the treatment of migraine has a long history. In the book of *Waitai Miyao* (*Arcane Essentials from the Imperial Library*), which was written during the Dang dynasty, it is recorded that GB-6 Xuanli on the side of the head is the meeting point of the Shaoyang Meridian and Yangming Meridian of both the hand and the foot.

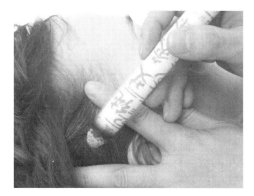

Figure 3.23 Moxibustion

Apply three moxa cones three times to treat febrile diseases, outer canthus pain, tinnitus, or sneezing.

MOXIBUSTION WITH A MOXA STICK

Moxibustion with a moxa stick involves igniting one end of the moxa stick and letting it smoke at a certain distance over the acupoint. The commonly used moxa sticks are pure moxa sticks or medicated moxa sticks. Moxibustion methods include circling moxibustion (moving moxa stick in a circular motion), and "sparrow-pecking" moxibustion (moving moxa stick vertically up and down).

Acupoints: GB-8 Shuaigu, ST-8 Touwei, BL-62 Shenmai, KI-6 Zhaohai, LU-7 Lieque, SI-3 Houxi, GB-41 Zulinqi, plus:

- EX-HN-3 Yintang and GB-14 Yangbai for pain on the forehead

- BL-10 Tianzhu and GB-20 Fengchi for pain on the back of the head

- DU-20 Baihui for pain on the apex of the head (Figure 3.24).

Notes: The main acupoints are confluence points of the eight extraordinary meridians. They regulate qi and blood, both in the regular meridian itself and in the extraordinary meridians. Apply moxibustion on the acupoints, depending on the patient's symptoms, to warm the meridians, remove blood stasis, and treat the cause of migraine. This method is suitable for treating migraine with patterns of phlegm turbidity, blood stasis, and coldness. Do not use this method for migraine due to yin deficiency with yang hyperactivity or ascendant hyperactivity of liver yang.

Manipulation: Ignite one end of the pure moxa stick and aim it towards one acupoint at a distance of 1–2cm from the skin. Adjust the distance according to the patient's sensation and changes to the skin. The patient should feel warm, but not burning, pain. Hold the moxa stick still when the patient feels warm and comfortable. Apply moxa first over the main acupoints, and then over the combined acupoints.

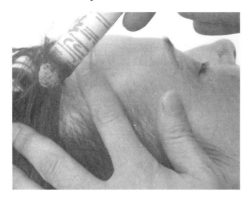

*Figure 3.24 Acupoints for
moxibustion with moxa stick*

Duration of treatment: Use moxa for 10–15 minutes each time, until the skin become slightly red. Apply moxa for 20 minutes for severe cases of migraine. The treatment is given once a day, and ten times forms a course of treatment.

MOXA CONE MOXIBUSTION

Moxa cone moxibustion uses pieces of moxa wool of various sizes, which are either placed directly on acupoints, or held over quantities of medical herbs placed on the skin, to treat the disease (respectively direct moxibustion and indirect moxibustion).

Direct moxibustion includes scarring and non-scarring moxibustion. The procedure and effect of the two methods are different.

Ginger (see below) is always used in indirect moxibustion.

Direct moxibustion

In direct moxibustion the ignited moxa cone is placed directly on the acupoint. The method comprises *scarring* and *non-scarring* moxibustion.

In *scarring* moxibustion the moxa cone is placed directly on the skin and causes blistering. This strong stimulation is good for severe cold blockage and pain. It strengthens the body's resistance to disease.

In *non-scarring* moxibustion the moxa cone is removed when the patient feels pain. This mild stimulation only reddens the skin without causing blisters. It is used to dispel cold, warm meridians, and improve microcirculation in the head. This moxibustion, as the name indicates, does not leave a scar. It is used mainly on the head or face, or on patients with low pain tolerance. Non-scarring moxibustion is used instead of direct moxibustion on the head to treat migraine.

Acupoints: SJ-23 Sizhukong, EX-HN-5 Taiyang, GB-14 Yangbai, GB-3 Shangguan, ST-8 Touwei (Figure 3.25).

Notes: This method directly treats the affected area. It achieves instant pain relief for migraine at the acute stage. It improves local qi and blood circulation and treats the cause of headache. However, direct moxibustion may leave scarring on the face, so be careful when using this method, and always check the patient's response. This method is suitable for treating migraine due to phlegm turbidity, blood stasis, and deficiency-cold.

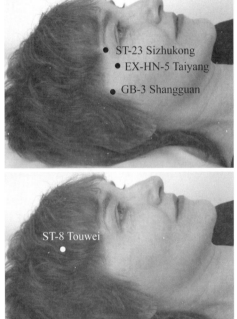
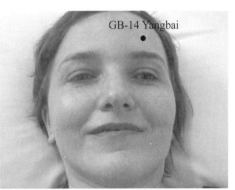
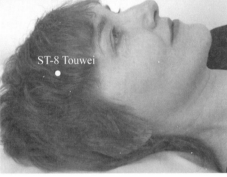

Figure 3.25 Acupoints for moxa cone moxibustion (direct)

Manipulation: Ignite a moxa cone the size of a lotus seed and place it on the acupoint. Remove the moxa cone when it is half to two-thirds burnt or the patient feels pain. Take another moxa cone and ignite it; place moxa on two acupoints simultaneously. Apply moxibustion treatment on five acupoints.

Duration of treatment: Use a series of 3–5 ignited moxa cones on one acupoint, to produce reddening of the skin without blistering. The treatment is given once a day, and ten times forms a course of treatment.

Indirect moxibustion

Indirect moxibustion, or partition moxibustion, is done by placing some materials, usually drugs, between the smouldering moxa cone and the skin. The usual form of indirect moxibustion comprises ginger moxibustion, salt moxibustion, garlic moxibustion, and fu zi (aconite root) moxibustion. The effect differs according to the substance used: for example, ginger moxibustion is good for warming meridians, dissipating cold, warming the middle, and arresting vomiting; salt moxibustion is used to warm the kidneys, assist yang, and restore yang to prevent from collapse; garlic moxibustion is used to draw out toxins and expel pus.

The main inducing factor for migraine is cold, which hinders qi and blood circulation, and so ginger moxibustion is used to warm the meridians. The ginger juice has little effect on the skin and does not cause blistering or scarring. It is suitable to be used for moxibustion on the head or the face.

Acupoints: SJ-22 Erheliao, GB-8 Shuaigu (Figure 3.26).

Notes: Migraine is closely related to qi and blood disorder. The pain is caused by cold in qi and blood. Ginger moxibustion uses moxa to warm the meridians and fresh ginger to warm the middle and dissipate cold, and SJ-22 Erheliao, the meeting point of the Sanjiao Meridian, Gallbladder Meridian, and Small Intestine Meridian, is used to warm the meridians and relieve pain. This method is used for migraine due to phlegm turbidity and blood stasis. It is commonly used to treat migraine due to external contraction of wind, cold, and dampness.

Manipulation: Cut fresh ginger into thin, coin-shaped slices. Ask the patient to lie on his side. Disinfect the acupoint in the normal way. Put a fresh ginger slice on SJ-22 Erheliao and put a peanut-sized moxa cone on top of the ginger slice to perform moxibustion.

Duration of treatment: Change the moxa cone when it is burnt out after three times. The treatment is given once a day, and ten times forms a course of treatment.

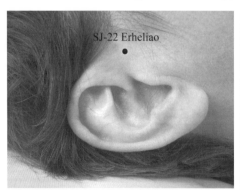 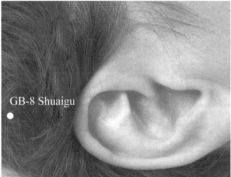

Figure 3.26 Acupoints for moxa cone moxibustion (indirect)

Lamp moxibustion

Lamp moxibustion is the method of dipping a piece of Dengxincao (*medulla junci*) in sesame oil, igniting it, and using it to rapidly moxa the acupoint. The quick stimulation is effective in dispersing wind, releasing exterior wind, and moving qi to relieve pain.

Acupoints: BL-2 Cuanzhu, ST-8 Touwei, GB-20 Fengchi, Ashi points (Figure 3.27).

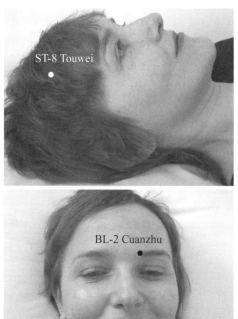
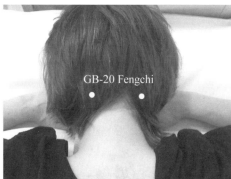
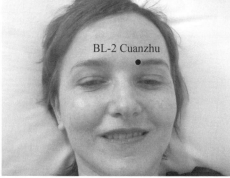

Figure 3.26 Acupoints for lamp moxibustion

Notes: This method leaves small blisters on the skin. Prick the blisters with the acupuncture needle and squeeze the liquid out. (Be careful not break the skin.) Disinfect the treated area to prevent infection. There will be no scar once the epidermis is shed. This method of moxibustion is commonly used to treat migraine due to external contraction of wind, cold, and dampness, or phlegm turbidity obstructing collaterals. Beware of giving this treatment to patients who scar easily.

Manipulation: Hold one end of a piece of Dengxincao (*medulla junci*) between the thumb and index finger. Dip it in sesame oil, ignite it, and rapidly moxa several acupoints. On the first treatment you will hear the sound of the ignited Dengxincao (*medulla junci*) touching the skin.

Duration of treatment: Moxibustion is given 3–5 times on each acupoint. The treatment is given every other day, and ten times forms a course of treatment.

Section II Other Acupuncture Therapies

Fire needle therapy

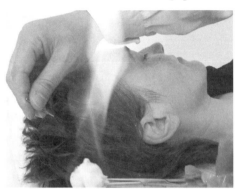

Figure 3.28 Fire needle therapy

Fire needling is done by heating a specially made needle until it is red-hot, and rapidly inserting it into the body to treat disease (Figure 3.28). In the book of *Huangdi Neijing: Miraculous Pivot, Discussion on Official Needling Technique* it is recorded that fire needling means to puncture with a heated needle to treat Bi syndromes. fire needling directly activates meridian qi by means of the heat of the needle. It promotes qi and blood circulation, warms meridians, dissipates cold, dredges meridians, and activates collaterals. fire needling also burns the sinews to dredge meridians. The stagnated blood is removed from the body through the needling holes.

Two points should be noted when using fire needling to treat migraine. First, the acupoint location needs to be accurate, and the fire needling acupoints should be no more than 4–6 each time, due to the pain caused by the treatment. Second, search for the tender point for the treatment, especially during a headache attack.

Acupoints: Ashi points, ST-8 Touwei (on the affected side), GB-8 Shuaigu (on the affected side), SJ-4 Yangchi, GB-40 Qiuxu (Figure 3.29).

Notes:

- Local points, such as Ashi points, ST-8 Touwei, GB-8 Shuaigu, are used to dredge qi and blood of the meridian.

- SJ-4 Yangchi and GB-40 Qiuxu are source points of the Triple Energizer Meridian and the Gallbladder Meridian respectively.

- It is normal for the skin to be red, burning, or slightly swollen after fire needling treatment. It recovers in several days without treatment.

- Avoid water contacting the puncture holes within 24 hours, to prevent infection.

- This method is suitable for migraine due to external contraction, phlegm-turbidity, blood stasis, or qi and blood deficiency. fire needling is effective in treating severe headache.

- Diabetic patients should not receive this treatment.

Manipulation: Disinfect the area to be treated in the normal way. Hold the ignited alcohol lamp with the left hand, and the needle with the right hand. Heat the needle in the outer region of the flame until it becomes red-hot, then white-hot. Prick quickly on the acupoint to a depth of between 0.2cm and 0.3cm. Withdraw the needle quickly and press it with dry, sterilized cottons balls soaked in iodine.

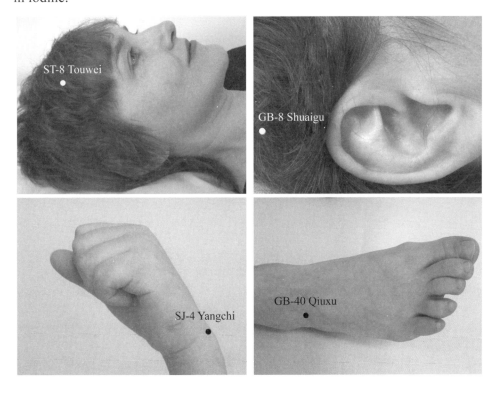

Figure 3.29 Acupoints for fire needle therapy

Duration of treatment: Treatment is given every other day during the attack stage, and once a week during remission, and ten times forms a course of treatment.

Dermal needle therapy

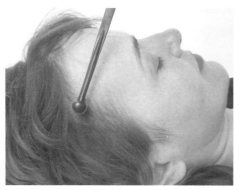 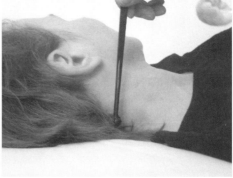

Figure 3.30 Dermal needle therapy

Dermal needle therapy is a multi-needle shallow puncture method, in which the area or acupoint is tapped with the dermal needle (Figure 3.30). It activates meridian function and regulates the qi and blood of Zang-Fu organs in order to treat or prevent disease.

Dermal needle therapy is based on cutaneous region theory. The cutaneous region is the first defensive system of the body and reveals the earliest symptoms of a disease. Meridians and the Zang-Fu organs are connected by the cutaneous region, so diseases can be transmitted deeper from the surface of the body, or internal disorders can orginate from the external region. According to this theory, puncturing certain acupoints, areas, or positive reaction points on the skin can dredge the meridians as well as harmonize qi and blood, as recorded in the book of *Huangdi Neijing*: *Miraculous Pivot, Discussion on Official Needling Technique*. It is recorded that half-needling means to insert the needle shallowly and withdraw the needle quickly. The needle should not penetrate deeply. The stimulation is just on the cutaneous region. The book of *Huangdi Neijing*: *Plain Questions, Discussion on Skin Divisions* records that the divisions (or the distribution) of the collaterals of the 12 channels are all divisions of the skin. So all diseases start from the body hair and skin.

Acupoints: ST-8 Touwei, GB-20 Fengchi, DU-20 Baihui (Figure 3.31).

Notes: Tapping the migraine-related acupoints activates blood, dredges collaterals, dispels wind, and dissipates cold. It relieves headache by activating qi and blood circulation and regulating related Zang-Fu function. The punctured points should not come in contact with water for at least 24 hours. Patients should not receive this therapy if there is trauma or ulcer on the skin. Patients with a tendency to bleed heavily should also not receive this treatment. This therapy is suitable for all types of migraine, especially migraine due to blood stasis.

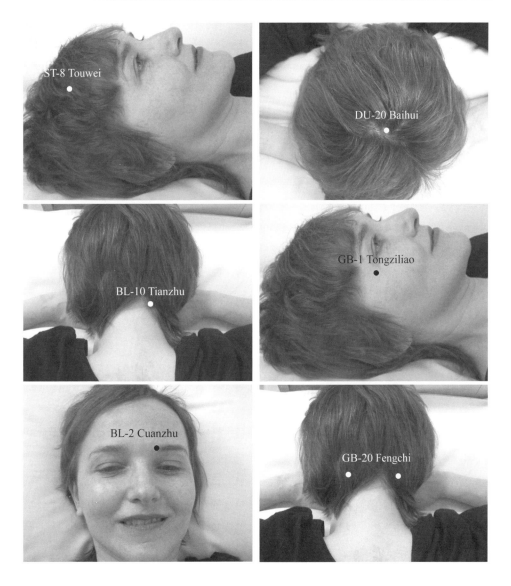

Figure 3.31 Acupoints for dermal needle therapy

Manipulation: Disinfect the skin of the area to be treated in the normal way. Hold the needle with the right hand and tap along the Gallbladder Meridian from the outer canthus of the eye, from GB-1 Tongziliao to GB-20 Fengchi. Then tap along the Bladder Meridian from BL-2 Cuanzhu to BL-10 Tianzhu. Tap the skin with medium stimulation, about 3–4 times at each point and at intervals of 1–1.5cm. Tap the skin to produce mild bleeding, for severe headache.

Duration of treatment: The treatment is given once a day, with ten times forming a course of treatment.

Acupoint injection therapy

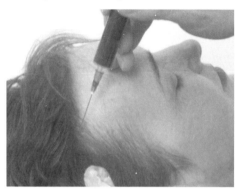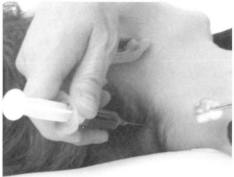

Figure 3.32 Acupoint injection therapy

Hydro-acupuncture, or acupoint injection therapy, is a new therapy which is based on the combination of modern medicine and acupuncture. This treatment injects Chinese medicine or modern pharmaceutical drugs into acupoints to improve body function and treat disease (Figure 3.32). It confers the effects of both acupuncture and medicine. This therapy activates both meridians and acupoints.

The two main factors in acupoint injection therapy are the acupoints and medicine that is injected.

SINGLE ACUPOINT INJECTION THERAPY

The main therapeutic effect of single acupoint injection therapy is caused by the medicine injected. The point is to make the medicine effective quickly and directly. This therapy is well accepted, as it is effective and requires few points.

Acupoints: GB-20 Fengchi (Figure 3.33).

Medicine: A mixture of 0.5mg Vitamin B_{12} and 2ml 2 percent lidocaine hydrochloride; or a mixture of 2ml ligustrazine hydrochloride for injection and 2ml lidocaine hydrochloride.

Notes: GB-20 Fengchi is at the superficial anatomical location where the greater occipital nerve exits from the skull. It is important for improving the blood supply to the brain. Sometimes there is pain or distension on the acupoint after the injection. It will disappear in 4–12 hours, without treatment. Check the quality of the medicine before injection to avoid side-effects. A skin test should be given, before the treatment, for patients with a drug-allergic history. This method is suitable for all types of migraine.

Manipulation: Draw medicine into a 5ml syringe. Disinfect the skin in the normal way. Insert the needle in the direction of the contralateral eyeball, to a depth of about 1 cun. Check that there is no bleeding on withdrawing the syringe when qi arrives, then inject 2ml medicine slowly into the point. Withdraw the needle and press the point with a dry cotton ball for one minute.

Duration of treatment: The treatment is given every other day, and five times forms a course of treatment.

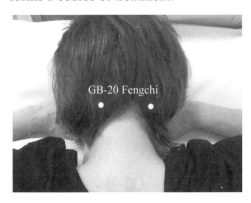

Figure 3.33 Acupoints for single acupoint injection therapy

CHINESE MEDICINE INJECTION THERAPY

Syndrome differentiation is used in the selection of both acupoints and drugs in Chinese medicine injection therapy. Acupoints are mainly selected according to visceral syndrome differentiation, and also combined with meridian pattern differentiation. (The Shaoyang Meridian is the one mainly involved.) Drugs are selected to treat qi stagnation and blood stasis, or phlegm accumulation due to qi deficiency. The commonly used Chinese medicine preparations are Danggui (*Radix angelicae sinensis*), Danshen (*Radix et rhizoma salviae miltiorrhizae*), Honghua (*Flos carthami*), and Huangqi (*Radix astragali*). They are effective at moving qi, activiting blood, nourishing blood, and dredging channels.

Acupoints:

- *Wind-dampness pattern*: GB-20 Fengchi, LI-4 Hegu, ST-8 Touwei (Figure 3.34).

- *Liver-yang pattern*: GB-5 Xuanlu, GB-4 Hanyan, LR-3 Taichong (Figure 3.35).

- *Phlegm-dampness pattern*: DU-23 Shangxing, ST-40 Fenglong, BL-20 Pishu (Figure 3.36).

- *Kidney-deficiency pattern*: DU-20 Baihui, BL-23 Shenshu, SP-6 Saoyinjiao (Figure 3.37).

Medicine: 5ml compound *Salviae miltiorrhizae*.

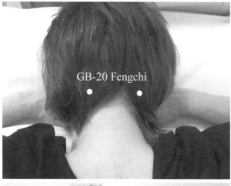

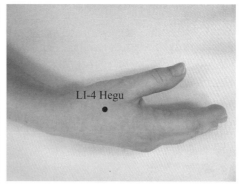

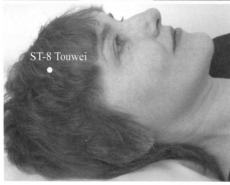

Figure 3.34 Acupoints for Chinese medicine injection therapy (wind dampness)

Notes:

- *wind-dampness pattern*: GB-20 Fengchi, LI-4 Hegu, ST-8 Touwei are used to expel wind, dissipate cold, resolve dampness, and dredge collaterals.

- *Liver-yang pattern*: GB-5 Xuanlu, GB-4 Hanyan, LR-3 Taichong are used to pacify the liver, descend adverse qi, subdue yang, and extinguish wind.

- *Phlegm-dampness pattern*: DU-23 Shangxing, ST-40 Fenglong, BL-20 Pishu are used to resolve phlegm, decrease turbidity, dredge collaterals, and relieve pain.

- *Kidney-deficiency pattern*: DU-20 Baihui, BL-23 Shenshu, SP-6 Sanyinjiao are used to nourish yin, tonify the kidneys, dredge collaterals, and relieve pain.

Meridian pattern differentiation is also used in the treatment. Acupoints are used from the Shaoyang Meridian, Yangming Meridian and Taiyang Meridian (mainly from the Shaoyang Meridian). The effect is strengthened by using compound *Salviae miltiorrhizae*, which is good at nourishing and activating blood to dredge collaterals.

Manipulation: Disinfect the skin in the normal way. Draw the medicine into a 5ml syringe. Insert the needle into the subcutaneous tissue. Check that there is no bleeding on withdrawing the syringe, then inject 1.5ml medicine into each point.

Duration of treatment: The treatment is given every other day, and 20 times forms a course of treatment.

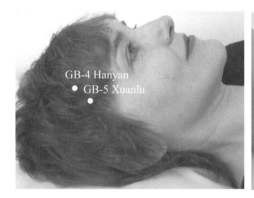
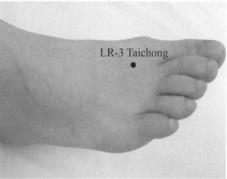

Figure 3.35 Acupoints for Chinese medicine injection therapy (liver yang)

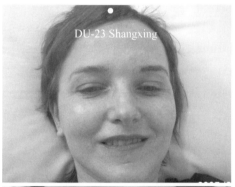
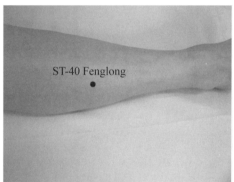

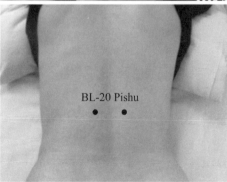

Figure 3.36 Acupoints for Chinese medicine injection therapy (phlegm dampness)

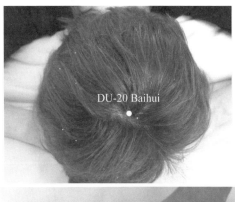

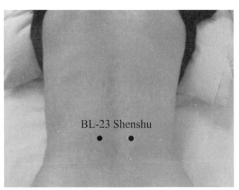

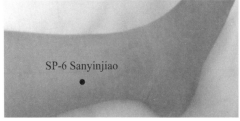

Figure 3.37 Acupoints for Chinese medicine injection therapy (kidney-deficiency)

MODERN MEDICINE INJECTION THERAPY

Modern medicine preparations are used mainly to nourish or stimulate the nervous system with direct and instant effect. However, some side-effects will also be presented as a result of using this method.

Acupoints: EX-HN-5 Taiyang, GB-5 Xuanlu, GB-8 Shuaigu, Ashi points (Figure 3.38).

Medicine: A mixture of 2ml Vitamin B_1 and 2 ml Vitamin B_{12}.

Notes: Acupoints selected in this method are commonly used in treating migraine. The injected Vitamin B_1 and Vitamin B_{12} are medicine to nourish the nerves. This method relieves pain for persistent, severe migraine cases.

Manipulation: Disinfect the skin in the normal way. Draw the medicine into a 5ml syringe. Rapidly insert the needle into the subcutaneous tissue. Check that there is no bleeding on withdrawing the syringe, then inject 1ml medicine into each point.

Duration of treatment: The treatment is given every other day, and five times forms a course of treatment.

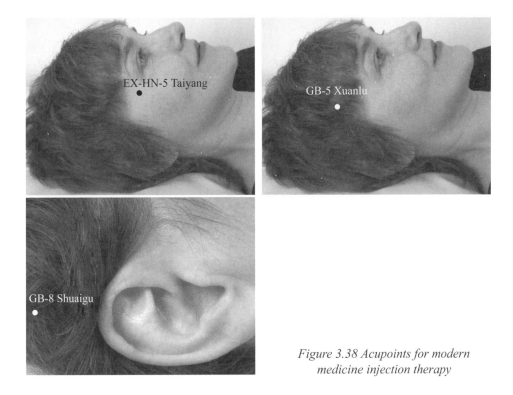

Figure 3.38 Acupoints for modern medicine injection therapy

Acupoint application therapy

In acupoint application therapy a certain drug, or mixture of several drugs, is applied on a specific acupoint to treat disease. It achieves the combined effect of both meridian and drug stimulation. The drug is absorbed by the skin without pricking the acupoint. This method is slow to take effect. However, there is no trauma or pain. It is well accepted by patients.

Acupoint selection for acupoint application therapy is similar to acupuncture. The applied drugs are mainly herbal medicine, which is selected according to syndrome differentiation.

Acupoints: EX-HN-5 Taiyang, GB-20 Fengchi, SJ-23 Sizhukong (Figure 3.39).

Medicine: Chenpi (*Pericarpium citri reticulatae*), Qianghuo (*Rhizoma et radix notopterygii*), Baizhi (*Radix angelicae dahuricae*), and Shengjiang (*Rhizoma zingiberis recens*).

Notes:

- EX-HN-5 Taiyang and GB-20 Fengchi are key points in treating headache.

- Most migraine patients feel discomfort or distension around the eyes before or during headache attack. SJ-23 Sizhukong, a Shaoyang Meridian acupoint, is an important acupoint in the eye area.

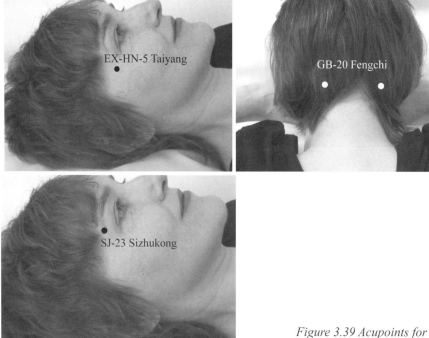

Figure 3.39 Acupoints for acupoint application therapy

- The region of GB-20 Fengchi is hairy, and the application easily falls off, so shave the area before therapy, or rub it with alcohol repeatedly and stick the application on when the alcohol has dried. This method is suitable for patients who are afraid of needles. Patients with skin allergy should not receive this therapy.

Manipulation: Prepare fresh ginger juice. Mix Chenpi (*Pericarpium citri reticulatae*), Qianghuo (*Rhizoma et radix notopterygii*) and Baizhi (*Radix angelicae dahuricae*) in proportions of 1:2:2. Pound into a powder and mix it with the fresh ginger juice. Make the mixture into a herbal medicine cake 1.5cm in diameter and 0.5cm high. Disinfect the skin in the normal way. Stick the herbal medicine cake onto acupoint with tape.

Duration of treatment: The herbal medicine cake is applied for 6–8 hours. The treatment is given once every three days, ten times forms a course of treatment.

Section III Combined Therapy

Many types of acupuncture therapy have been described in this book. In clinical practice, these methods are usually combined. The commonly used therapy combinations are as follows.

Filiform needling with moxibustion

The combination of filiform needling and moxibustion is used to warm meridians and combine nourishment with reduction. Applying moxibustion after acupuncture activates Shaoyang Meridian qi, as well as warming meridians and dissipating cold. This therapy is suitable for migraine due to qi deficiency, disorder, or congealing cold in the Shaoyang Meridian, or weak constitution.

Acupoints: EX-HN-5 Taiyang, ST-8 Touwei, GB-17 Zhengying, GB-8 Shuaigu, DU-20 Baihui, LI-4 Hegu, LR-3 Taichong, SJ-10 Tianjing, SJ-3 Zhongzhu, GB-43 Xiaxi (Figure 3.40).

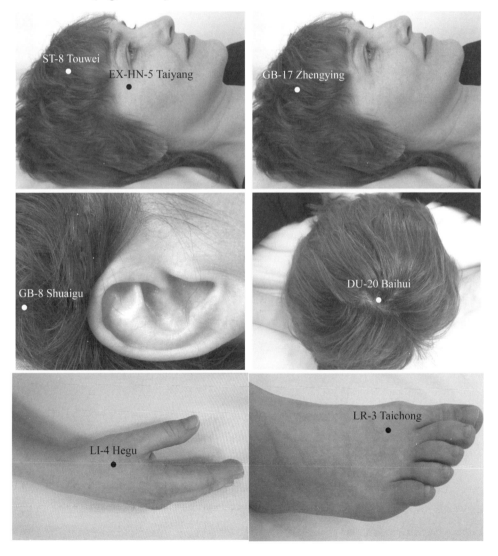

Figure 3.40 Acupoints for filiform needling with moxibustion

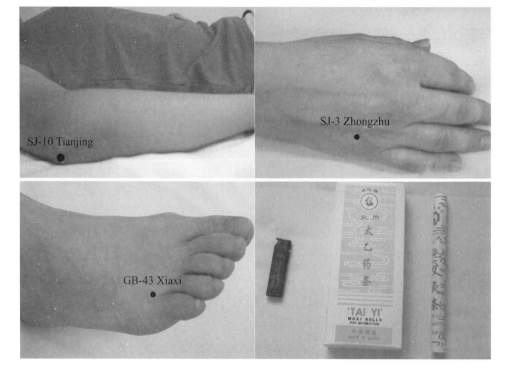

Figure 3.40 Acupoints for filiform needling with moxibustion cont.

Manipulation: Disinfect the skin in the normal way. Insert 1.5 cun filiform needles to acupoints LI-4 Hegu, LR-3 Taichong, and other acupoints, from the upper part of the body to the lower part of the body. Twirl the needles with neutral reinforcement and reduction when qi arrives.

Ignite a moxa stick and give mild moxibustion on each acupoint following the order of needling. Patients should feel warm, but not burning, pain during moxibustion. The skin becomes red. Remove the needles after moxibustion.

Duration of treatment: Needles should be retained for 30 minutes. Manipulate the needle every ten minutes. The treatment is given every other day, and ten times forms a course of treatment.

Filiform needling with fire needling

In this therapy fire needling is used to dredge local meridian qi and activate qi and blood, and filiform needling is used to regulate the meridian qi of the Shaoyang Meridian. It is suitable for persistent, severe migraine. The migraine is caused by cold but lacks effective treatment. The cold invades the meridian and leads to qi and blood stagnation. This therapy is effective in treating migraine due to blood stasis.

Local acupoints are mainly used in fire needling. The key acupoints in treating headache are EX-HN-5 Taiyang and Ashi points. fire needle on DU-20 Baihui is used to lift yang qi in the human body and maintain the head as the meeting area of all yang. GB-20 Fengchi is the connection between head and neck. It plays an important role in supplying qi and blood to the head. (Modern research shows that stimulating this acupoint improves the blood and oxygen supply to the head.)

Filiform needle acupoints: SJ-5 Waiguan, SJ-3 Zhongzhu, GB-41 Zulinqi, GB-43 Xiaxi (Figure 3.41).

Fire needle acupoints: GB-20 Fengchi, EX-HN-5 Taiyang, DU-20 Baihui, Ashi points (Figure 3.42).

Manipulation: Disinfect the skin in the normal way. Hold the ignited alcohol lamp with the left hand, and the needle with the right hand. Heat the needle body in the outer region of the flame until the needle becomes red-hot, then white-hot.

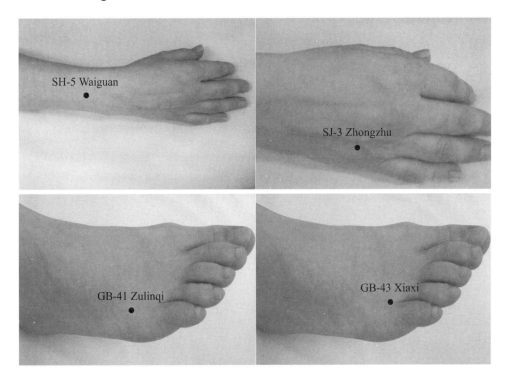

Figure 3.41 Acupoints for filiform needling with fire needling (filiform needle)

Disinfect the acupoint in the normal way. Use 1.5 cun needles for the treatment. Prick quickly on the acupoint to a depth of 0.2–0.3cm. Withdraw the needle quickly. Prick each acupoint two or three times. Manipulate the needles with neutral reinforcement and reduction when qi arrives. The needling sensation for GB-20 Fengchi should be a warm sensation spreading upwards, or towards the ear. The sensation of EX-HN-5 Taiyang and tender points should be heat, numbness, or distension spreading around the head. Little red spots or bleeding will be caused by fire needling. Press the punctures with dry, sterilized cotton balls.

Duration of treatment: Needles are retained for 30 minutes. Manipulate the needles every ten minutes. The treatment is given every other day, and ten times forms a course of treatment.

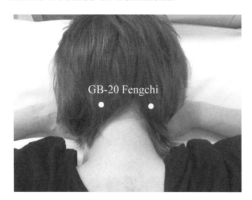

Figure 3.42 Acupoints for filiform needling with fire needling (fire needle)

Filiform needling with acupoint injection

Filiform needling is used to regulate meridian qi. The injected drugs are used to nourish blood, dispel wind, activate the blood, and dredge the meridians. Apply acupuncture first to regulate meridian qi. Then inject the recommended drug on GB-20 Fengchi to treat migraine.

The acupoint selection combines Shaoyang Meridian acupoints with local acupoints to treat both the symptoms and the cause of headache. GB-20 Fengchi is an acupoint for activating blood and dispelling wind. Injection on this acupoint improves the blood supply to the head.

Acupoints: LI-4 Hegu, LR-3 Taichong, DU-20 Baihui, EX-HN-5 Taiyang, ST-8 Touwei, SJ-10 Tianjing, SJ-3 Zhongzhu, GB-43 Xiaxi (Figure 3.43).

Medicine: 2ml compound *Angelicae sinensis*.

Manipulation: Disinfect the acupoint in the normal way. Use 1.5 cun needles for the treatment. Twirl the needles with neutral reinforcement and reduction when qi arrives.

Disinfect GB-20 Fengchi on both sides after removing needles. Draw the medicine into a 2ml syringe. Insert the needle quickly into the acupoint, directed toward the contralateral eyeball. Check that there is no bleeding on withdrawing the syringe when qi arrives, then inject 1ml medicine into the point. Perform the same procedure on the other side.

Duration of treatment: Needles are retained for 30 minutes. Manipulate the needles every ten minutes. The treatment is given every other day, and ten times forms a course of treatment.

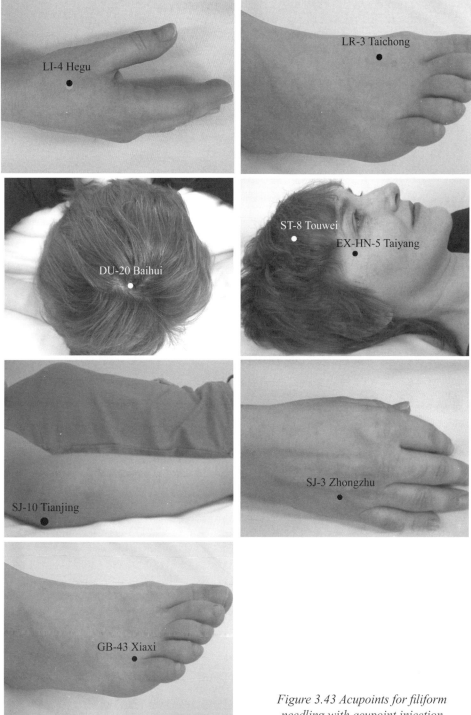

Figure 3.43 Acupoints for filiform
needling with acupoint injection

Filiform needling with cupping

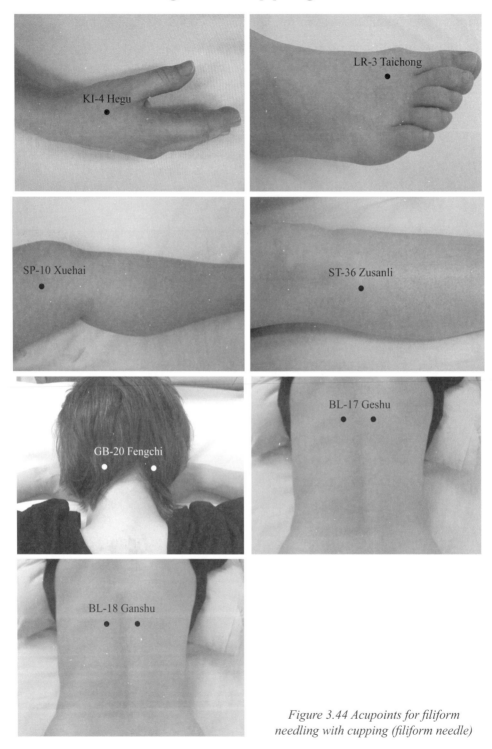

Figure 3.44 Acupoints for filiform needling with cupping (filiform needle)

This is a very common combination in clinical practice. Acupuncture regulates meridian qi, and cupping regulates Zang-Fu function. This therapy is suitable for migraine due to blood stasis, or migraine related to Zang-Fu dysfunction.

Acupoints for filiform needling: LI-4 Hegu, LR-3 Taichong, SP-10 Xuehai, ST-36 Zusanli, GB-20 Fengchi, BL-17 Geshu, BL-18 Ganshu (Figure 3.44).

Acupoints for cupping: GB-20 Fengchi, BL-17 Geshu, BL-18 Ganshu (Figure 3.45).

Manipulation: Ask the patient either to sit or to lie on his side. Disinfect the acupoint in the normal way. Insert a needle into GB-20 Fengchi, with the tip directed towards the contralateral eyeball. Position needles perpendicularly on the other acupoints. Place cups on GB-20 Fengchi, BL-17 Geshu and BL-18 Ganshu. Remove the cups when stagnated marks appear on the skin.

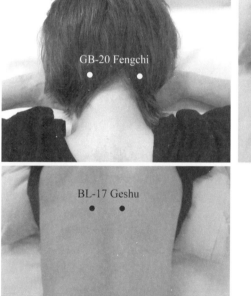

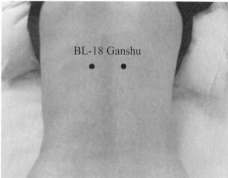

Figure 3.45 Acupoints for filiform needling with cupping (cupping)

Duration of treatment: Needles are retained for 30 minutes; cups for ten minutes. Remove the cups earlier if there are too many stagnated marks. The treatment is given every other day, and ten times forms a course of treatment.

Electric acupuncture with ear acupuncture

Acupuncture is used to regulate meridian qi on the head. The continuous wave of an electric stimulator is used instead of manual manipulation, to prolong the needling sensation. Ear acupuncture is used to directly adjust the sensory nerves of the head via the parasympathetic nerves. It also regulates related Zang-Fu organ function. This therapy treats the symptoms as well as the cause of the disease.

The acupoint selection on the body combines local acupoints and distal acupoints. Ear acupuncture is used to adjust nerve system, using points such as Shenmen, Sympathetic and Subcortex. Ear acupoints of the Forehead, Temples, and Occipital region are selected, depending on the location of pain. Liver and Gallbladder are used for the related Zang-Fu organ.

Acupoints: GB-20 Fengchi, GB-12 Wangu, LR-3 Taichong, BL-63 Jinmen, GB-41 Zulinqi (Figure 3.46).

Ear acupoints: Shenmen, Sympathetic, Subcortex, Liver, Gallbladder, Forehead, Temple, and Occipital (Figure 3.47).

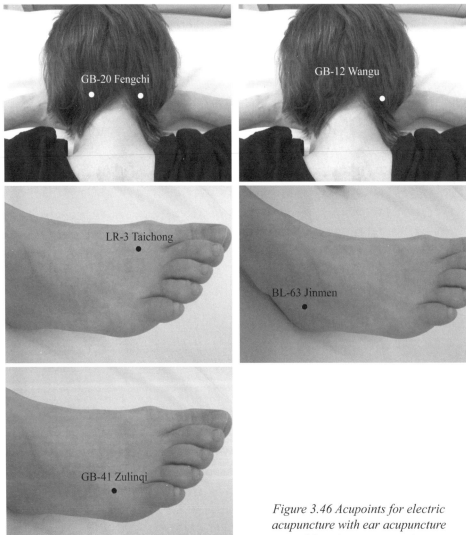

Figure 3.46 Acupoints for electric acupuncture with ear acupuncture (electric acupuncture)

Manipulation: Disinfect the acupoints in the normal way. Insert 1.5 cun filiform needles obliquely on GB-20 Fengchi and GB-12 Wangu. The needling sensation should be radiated to the forehead or EX-HN-5 Taiyang on the same side. The needle tip of GB-20 Fengchi should be aimed towards the contralateral eyeball. Position needles perpendicularly on other acupoints. Connect the needles to the electric stimulator with a continuous wave. Adjust the intensity and frequency according to the patient's tolerance.

Search for sensitive points on the ear after acupuncture treatment. Disinfect the ear routinely. Fix seeds of Wangbuliuxing (*semen vaccariae*) on the tender points with tape. Find the most painful points, which cause slight prickly pain on the ear.

Duration of treatment: Electric acupuncture is maintained for 30 minutes. The treatment is given every other day. Keep the seeds on the ear. Both ears are used alternately. Ten times forms a treating course.

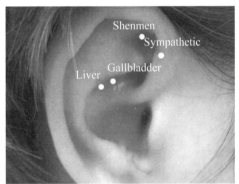 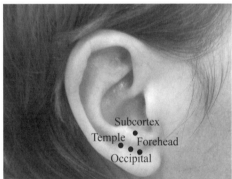

Figure 3.47 Acupoints for electric acupuncture with ear acupuncture (ear acupuncture)

Electric acupuncture with bloodletting therapy

This therapy uses fewer acupoints. It combines acupuncture, electric acupuncture, bloodletting, and cupping. The stimulation of this therapy is relatively strong. It is suitable for migraine due to blood stasis. Acupuncture is used to dredge the Shaoyang Meridian on the head. Bloodletting with cupping on BL-17 Geshu dispels stasis to promote regeneration, activate the blood, and dredge the meridians.

Acupoints: EX-HN-5 Taiyang, GB-20 Fengchi, GB-8 Shuaigu, SJ-3 Zhongzhu (Figure 3.48).

Bloodletting point: BL-17 Geshu (Figure 3.49).

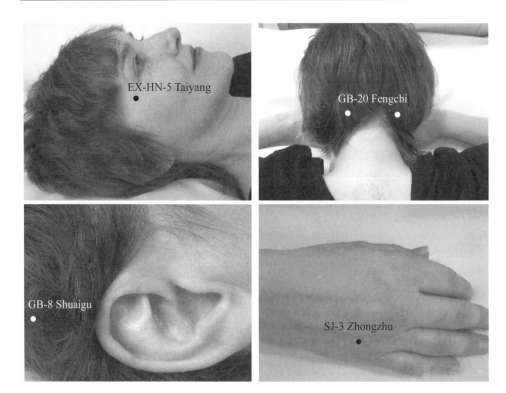

Figure 3.48 Acupoints for electric acupuncture with bloodletting (electric acupuncture)

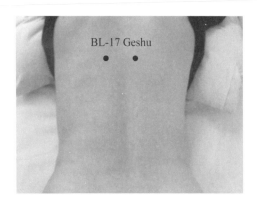

Figure 3.49 Acupoints for electric acupuncture with bloodletting (bloodletting)

Manipulation: Disinfect acupoints in the normal way. Insert 1.5 cun filiform needles on the acupoints. The needle tip of GB-20 Fengchi should be aimed towards the contralateral eyeball. Position needles perpendicularly on the other acupoints. Connect the needles to the electric stimulator with a continuous wave when qi arrives. Adjust the intensity and frequency according to the patients's tolerance.

After removing the needles, disinfect BL-17 Geshu and the surrounding skin with iodine. Prick the point superior, inferior, and lateral to BL-17 Geshu with a three-edged needle (or disposable injection needle). Cover the acupoint with a large cup to collect the blood. Disinfect the area after removing the cup.

Duration of treatment: Electric acupuncture is maintained for 30 minutes; cups are kept for ten minutes. The treatment is given every other day, and ten times forms a course of treatment.

Ear acupuncture with acupoint injection

Ear acupuncture is used to adjust autonomic nerves. Acupoint injection is used to nourish the blood, expel wind, activate the blood, and dredge the meridians. This method is suitable for all types of migraine. It is especially effective for patients during the attack phase when there is no specific cause or complex pattern. Ear acupuncture is used first, to relieve pain by the self-adjusting of the autonomic nerve. Then drugs are injected to treat the pain.

Ear acupoints: Shenmen, Subcortex, Liver, Forehead, and Occipital (Figure 3.50).

Acupoint injection: GB-34 Yanglingquan and Ashi points (Figure 3.51).

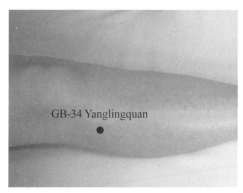

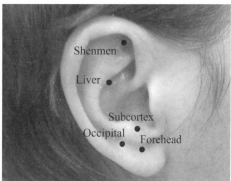

Figure 3.50 Acupoint for ear acupuncture with acupoint injection (ear acupuncture)

Figure 3.51 Acupoints for ear acupuncture with acupoint injection (acupoint injection)

Medicine: 2ml compound *Angelicae sinensis*.

Manipulation: Search for tender points on the ear. Disinfect the points in the normal way. Fix seeds of Wangbulinxing (*semen vaccariae*) on the tender points with tape. Find the most painful points, which cause slight prickly pain on the ear.

Disinfect GB-34 Yanglingquan and Ashi points. Draw the medicine into a 5ml syringe. Rapidly insert the needles into the acupoints. Check that there is no bleeding on withdrawing the syringe. Inject 1ml medicine into each point.

Duration of treatment: The treatment is given every other day, and ten times forms a course of treatment. Use both ears alternately.

Scalp acupuncture with acupoint injection

Scalp acupuncture is used to adjust the cortex function. Acupoint injection is used to improve microcirculation and increase the oxygen supply to the brain. This method is suitable for all types of migraine. It is especially effective for patients during the attack stage when there is no specific cause or complex pattern.

Stimulate the related regions with scalp acupunture to adjust cortex function and relieve pain. Then inject compound Ciwujia (*Radix et rhizoma seu caulis acanthopanacis senticosi*) on acupoints to improve the blood and oxygen supply to the head.

Scalp acupuncture: The *lower* two-fifths of the sensory area on the healthy side; foot motor area (Figure 3.52).

Acupoint injection: GB-20 Fengchi, GB-38 Yangfu, SJ-5 Waiguan (Figure 3.53).

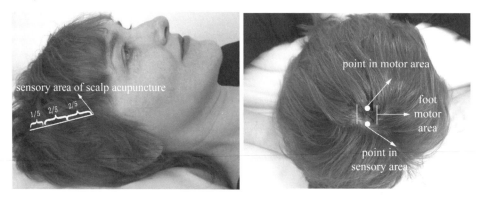

Figure 3.52 Acupoints for scalp acupuncture with acupoint injection (scalp acupuncture)

Medicine: 18ml compound Ciwujia (*Radix et rhizoma seu caulis acanthopanacis senticosi*).

Manipulation: Disinfect scalp points in the normal way. Insert 1.5 cun filiform needles into acupoints at an angle of 15–30 degrees. Needling resistance decreases when the needle arrives at the galea aponeurotica. Insert the needle 1 cun horizontally, with rapid twirling manipulation.

After removing the needles, disinfect the skin in the normal way. Draw 3ml medicine into a 5ml syringe. Insert the needle into the first acupoint. Check that there is no bleeding on withdrawing the syringe when qi arrives, then inject medicine into the point. Withdraw the needle and press the point with a dry cotton ball for two minutes. Follow the same procedure on the other two acupoints.

Duration of treatment: Needles are retained for 30 minutes. Manipulate the needles every ten minutes. The treatment is given every other day, and ten times forms a course of treatment.

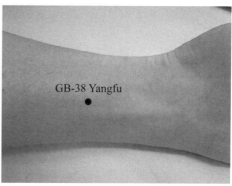

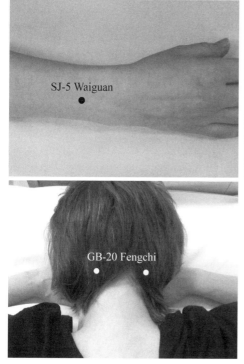

Figure 3.53 Acupoints for scalp acupuncture with acupoint injection (acupoint injection)

Bloodletting therapy with acupoint injection

The cause of migraine due to blood stasis is stagnated blood blocking meridians. Stagnated blood also hinders qi and blood circulation, and so the head is undernourished. The treatment is to prick for blood and eliminate stagnated blood. Drugs are injected to nourish and activate the blood via acupoints. Headache is relieved when the meridian is regulated.

Bloodletting points: EX-HN-5 Taiyang and Ashi points (Figure 3.54).

Acupoint injection: SJ-23 Sizhukong to GB-8 Shuaigu, GB-20 Fengchi (Figure 3.55).

Medicine: 4ml ligustrazine.

Manipulation: Disinfect the superficial veins around EX-HN-5 Taiyang in the normal way. Prick the collaterals with three-edged needle (or disposable injection needle). Prick the blood vessel wall superficially. Cover the pricking point with a cup for five minutes to collect 1–3ml blood. Search for tender or sensitive points in the pain region (usually nodules), or for obvious superficial veins. Disinfect the skin in the normal way. Prick each point with a three-edged needle (or disposable injection needle). Let the tip of the needle touch the nodule or prick the collaterals. Squeeze 0.5–2ml blood out of the point.

Disinfect the skin in the normal way. Draw the medicine into a 5ml syringe. Insert the needle into SJ-23 Sizhukong, then direct the tip of the needle slowly towards GB-8 Shuaigu after pricking the skin. Check that there is no bleeding on withdrawing the syringe when qi arrives. Inject 2ml medicine into the point while withdrawing the needle. Press the point with a dry cotton ball for two minutes to prevent bleeding.

Slowly insert the needle on GB-20 Fengchi with the tip towards the tip of the nose. Make the needling sensation radiate to EX-HN-5 Taiyang or obtain qi locally. Check that there is no bleeding on withdrawing the syringe. Inject 2ml medicine into the point. Withdraw the needle and press the point with a dry cotton ball for two minutes to prevent bleeding.

Duration of treatment: The treatment is given every other day, and seven times forms a course of treatment.

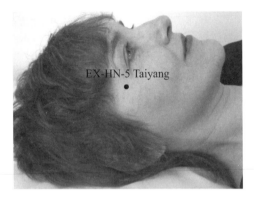

Figure 3.54 Acupoint for bloodletting therapy with acupoint injection (bloodletting)

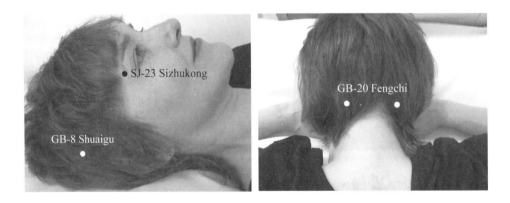

Figure 3.55 Acupoints for bloodletting therapy with acupoint injection (acupoint injection)

Filiform needling with fire needling and bloodletting therapy

Filiform needling is used to regulate the meridians. Fire needling is applied to warm the meridians. Bloodletting therapy aims to dispel stasis to promote regeneration. The stimulation is strong with both fire needling and bloodletting therapy. This method is suitable for migraine due to congealing cold within the meridians, blood stasis, and medium or severe persistent cases of migraine.

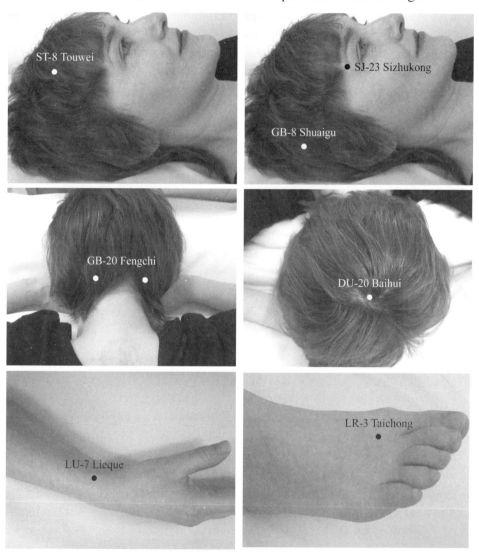

Figure 3.56 Acupoints for filiform
needling with fire needling and bloodletting therapy (filiform needle)

Filiform needle acupoints: ST-8 Touwei, SJ-23 Sizhukong to GB-8 Shuaigu, GB-20 Fengchi, DU-20 Baihui, LU-7 Lieque, LR-3 Taichong (Figure 3.56).

Fire needle acupoints: Ashi points.

Bloodletting points: EX-HN-5 Taiyang, EX-HN-1 Sishencong (Figure 3.57).

Manipulation: Disinfect the acupoints in the normal way. Use 1.5 cun needles for the treatment. Insert the needle horizontally on ST-8 Touwei. Penetrating needling is used from SJ-23 Sizhukong to GB-8 Shuaigu. Insert the needles perpendicularly on the other acupoints. Manipulate the needles with neutral reinforcement and reduction when qi arrives. Search for tender points after removing the needles. Apply routine disinfection on the area to be treated.

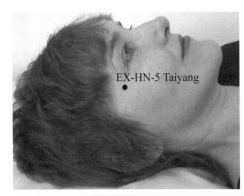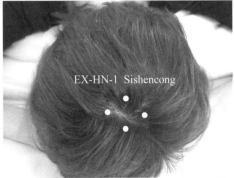

Figure 3.57 Acupoints for filiform needling with fire needling
and bloodletting therapy (bloodletting)

Holding the ignited alcohol lamp with the left hand, and the needle with the right hand, heat the needle body in the outer region of the flame until the needle becomes red-hot, then white-hot. Prick quickly on the acupoint to a depth of 0.2–0.3cm. Withdraw the needle quickly, and press the puncture hole with dry, sterile cotton balls. Disinfect the acupoint with iodine.

　　Disinfect EX-HN-5 Taiyang and EX-HN-1 Sishencong with iodine. Prick each acupoint with a three-edged needle (or disposable injection needle). Squeeze out some blood and press the pricking hole with dry, sterile cotton balls.

Duration of treatment: Needles are retained for 30 minutes. Manipulate the needles every ten minutes. The treatment is given every other day, and ten times forms a course of treatment.

Chapter *4*

Tuina Manipulation for Treating Migraine

Tuina manipulation is a traditional therapy with a long history. There were early records on Tuina in *Huangdi Neijing and Huangdi Qibo An mo Shi Juan*, and with the unremitting dedication of generations of medical scholars, Tuina manipulation has become a specific therapy with its own integrated theoretical system and diverse schools. The different schools of Tuina hold different views on the treatment of migraine, each possessing its own particular body of detailed information on specific acupoints and manipulations for treating the condition.

Section I Tuina Theory

Tuina manipulation is commonly used for treating migraine. It is readily acceptable to patients, because it is comfortable and has no traumatic effects. Basic theories on Tuina are outlined below.

Theory of Chinese medicine

Tuina manipulation is effective in treating migraine, as evidenced in the abundant clinical experience gained over thousands of years.

Proper manipulation contributes to soothing tendons and activating collaterals, regulating the qi mechanism, promoting circulation of qi and blood, improving the functioning of the Zang-Fu organs, and adjusting the balance of yin and yang. The symptoms of migraine can be relieved in the following ways.

REGULATING QI TO RELIEVE PAIN

Regulation of the qi mechanism moves qi and activates blood, soothes collaterals, nourishes the brain, and relieves headache. It is used mainly to relieve migraine caused by disturbance of qi movement.

ACTIVATING BLOOD TO RELIEVE PAIN

Activating blood helps to accelerate the circulation of qi and blood, eliminating blood stasis to relieve headache. It is mainly applied to relieve migraine caused by blood stasis and irregular blood supply.

ELIMINATING DAMPNESS TO RELIEVE PAIN

Eliminating humidity and retention of phlegm unblocks collaterals and channels, so that pain is relieved by normalized channelling of qi. It is mainly used to treat migraine induced by interior or exterior dampness, or phlegm retention blocking collaterals.

WARMING CHANNELS AND DISSIPATING COLD

Pain is relieved in the process of warming the channels and dissipating cold. It is mainly used to treat migraine caused by cold, damp chill, or phlegm retention blocking collaterals.

DISPELLING WIND TO RELIEVE PAIN

Dispelling wind, as well as activating blood, reflects the principle of "treating blood to treat wind, regulation of blood will dispel wind." It is used to treat migraine induced by exterior wind.

REPLENISHING QI AND ACTIVATING BLOOD

Replenishing qi activates normal blood flow, so that pain is relieved. It is mainly used to treat migraine that is caused by qi deficiency induced blood or qi deficiency induced stasis.

NOURISHING BLOOD TO RELIEVE PAIN

Nourishing the blood stimulates the supply of blood to the Zang-Fu organs, so that pain is relieved. It is mainly used to treat migraine induced by blood deficiency.

WARMING YANG AND DISPELLING COLD

Warming and tonifying yang qi to dispel interior cold warms the collaterals of the Zang-Fu organs, and promotes qi and blood supply to relieve pain. It is mainly used to treat migraine caused by a yang deficiency resulting from inner cold that blocks the collaterals, blood, and qi.

NOURISHING YIN

Nourishing kidney yin supplies abundant yin to relieve pain. It is used to relieve pain caused by lack of yin, which induces brain marrow.

Theory of Western medicine

According to Western medicine, the following results may be achieved by using Tuina to treat migraine.

REGULATING NERVE FUNCTION

Migraine is caused by abnormal nerve function and vasomotion. Tuina manipulation regulates the functioning of nerves and blood vessels, promotes cellular metabolism, increases tissue oxygenation, enhances cell viability, and improves blood supply and oxygen supply. At the same time, Tuina manipulation regulates the motions caused by the electronic charge in the cerebral cortex, improves cerebrovascular microcirculation, and regulates the functioning of nerve centers. Different manipulations should be applied on different therapeutic locations, to control excitability in the sympathetic nervous system, by increasing as well as decreasing excitability, in addition to adjusting nerve conduction. Migraine will be relieved as these aspects of nerve function return to normality.

REGULATING CIRCULATION

First of all, the effect of Tuina manipulation on blood vessels is manifested mainly as angiotelectasis, i.e. dilation of capillaries. Tuina manipulation causes a degree of protein disintegration, which produces histamine and, as a result, dilation of capillaries. This shows that Tuina manipulation not only increases angiotelectasis, but also enlarges the dimension of the capillary vessel, which enhances osmotic effect and increases blood flow, so that blood supply and the nutrition of local tissues are improved.

Second, when pressure is applied to acupoints, blood flow will be temporarily cut off if an artery is pressed in the direction of blood flow or nerve conduction. When pressure is released, blood will suddenly fill the location, and local circulation will be immediately improved.

Last, pressure and friction produced on the body surface by Tuina manipulation greatly consume and clean the lipoid from the blood vessel walls, to reduce vascular sclerosis, so that the flexibility of the blood vessel wall and the permeability of the blood vessel are improved, and peripheral resistance of blood flow is decreased.

RELEASING MUSCLE SPASM

Migraine usually accompanies muscular spasm in the neck region, and if muscular spasm is not relieved, migraine may be aggravated. Muscle spasm results from the contraction of muscles when local nerves are stimulated by abnormal signals. This is a spontaneous, protective response of the human body to prevent aggravation, but, unless effective measures are taken, muscle spasm stimulates nerves which in turn aggravate spasm and pain, forming a vicious circle. The purpose of Tuina is to release spasm, break the vicious circle, and restore the function of tissues. Tuina manipulation not only directly relaxes muscles, but also treats the causes of spasm, and restores balance to the body with its soothing action and relaxing effect.

ABSORBING PATHOLOGICAL PRODUCTS

Migraine impairs local blood circulation, and this gradually causes the deposit of pathologens such as 5-HTNA. These stimulate blood vessel walls, causing spasm, and then migraine is induced. When Tuina is applied, local blood circulation is improved, and the accelerated blood flow reduces or eliminates the pathologens, so that spasm of the blood vessels is relaxed, and migraine is also relieved.

Section II One-Finger-Pushing Manipulation

Summary

One-finger-pushing manipulation is one school of Tuina for preventing and treating disease. The practitioner uses thumb-pushing combined with grasping, rubbing, pressing, kneading, shaking, twisting, and other manipulations.

According to the theory of one-finger-pushing manipulation, the pathogenesis of migraine is that hyperactivity of ascendant liver yang and ascending counterflow of yang qi causes the hardening of blood channels and dysfunction of blood and qi circulation. Meanwhile, the mind is disturbed and mental activity irritated by the abnormal, upward reversal of yang qi, so that migraine is induced. Therefore, one-finger-pushing manipulation is applied to treat migraine, following the therapeutic principle of pacifying the liver and subduing yang, dredging channels, and activating collaterals, as well as soothing and relieving pain. Traditional channel point, extra point, and Ashi point manipulations are applied as well.

Treatment

Therapeutic principle: Dredging channels and activating collaterals, pacifying liver and subduing yang, soothing and relieving pain.

Manipulations: Pushing, grasping, wiping, hook-pushing, pressing, kneading, twisting.

Therapeutic area: EX-HN-3 Yintang, EX-HN-5 Taiyang, GB-4 Hanyan, BL-1 Jingming, frontal region, orbital region, GB-20 Fengchi, DU-16 Fengfu, DU-15 Yamen, SJ-17 Yifeng, urinary bladder meridian in the region of the nape, BL-18 Ganshu, SP-6 Sanyinjiao, costal regions.

Method: Apply one-finger push to the Bladder Meridian in the region of the nape; grasp GB-20 Fengchi and DU-16 Fengfu; press DU-15 Yamen (Figure 4.1); push EX-HN-3 Yintang and EX-HN-5 Taiyang; press GB-4 Hanyan and EX-HN-5 Taiyang; wipe the frontal and orbital region (Figure 4.2); hook-push the line from EX-HN-5 Taiyang to GB-20 Fengchi, grasping GB-20 Fengchi; press and knead SJ-17 Yifeng (Figure 4.3); press BL-1 Jingming; wipe the orbital region and EX-HN-3 Yintang; push BL-18 Ganshu; twist the costal regions and grasp SP-6 Sanyinjiao (Figure 4.4).

Duration of treatment: 2–5 minutes for each point, no more than 40 minutes for a complete treatment, once a day, 20 times forms a course of treatment.

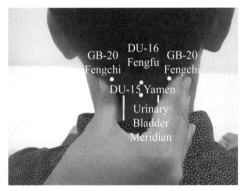 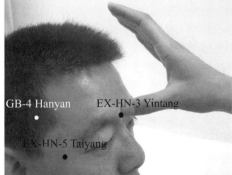

Figure 4.1 One-finger-pushing on the neck   *Figure 4.2 One-finger-pushing on the face*

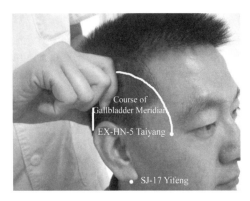

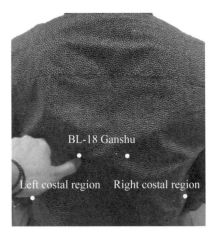

Figure 4.3 One-finger-pushing on the temples

Figure 4.4 One-finger-pushing on the body

Key points

PUSHING

Place the tip, the flank, and the tip of radialis of the thumb on the channel points or regions, relax the shoulder and elbow joints, and exert a constant force on the channels, points, and regions by continually swinging the wrist and flexing and extending thumb joint. Figure 4.2 illustrates the one-finger-pushing manipulation which is the key constituent of the one-finger-pushing schools.

Key: Relax the shoulder (relax the shoulder joint, without shrugging the shoulder); drop the elbow (relax the muscles of the upper limb, and lower the elbow below the wrist); drop the wrist (drop and flex the wrist, keeping the thumb vertical so as to be able to swing the wrist left and right); straighten the thumb (position the tip, the flank, and the tip of radialis of the thumb on the treatment area, and exert mild pressure); and soften the palm (make a hollow fist, keeping the fingers away from the palm and the thumb vertical, and the radialis of the middle joint of the index finger against the flank or joint of the thumb so as to stabilize the joint activity).

GRASPING

Applying even force through the thumb and the index finger and middle finger, or the thumb and the other four fingers, grasp, alternately, gently and then firmly. When grasping, the wrist can be rotated slightly in order to increase stimulus and achieve better effects. This is also called one-finger-grasping manipulation (Figure 4.5).

WIPING

Place the flanks of the thumbs in contact with the surface of the body, and do the up–down, left–right, or curved manipulation, sliding the thumbs apart and back together again (Figure 4.6).

Key: Keep the flanks of the thumbs firmly on the skin, and apply the linear or curved direction of manipulation, with the other four fingers to either side of the treated area. The force should be firm but not heavy, gentle but not superficial.

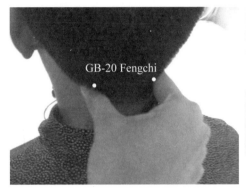

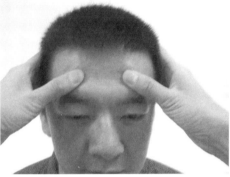

Figure 4.5 Grasping (one-finger-pushing manipulation)

Figure 4.6 Wiping (one-finger-pushing manipulation)

HOOK-PUSHING

Flex the fingers like a hook, and perform the hook-pushing manipulation at EX-HN-5 Taiyang, then on the temporal region, and at BL-9 Yuzhen, along the Gallbladder Meridian. Then the manipulation is divided into two parts:

- First, do the wiping manipulation with the index finger from BL-9 Yuzhen to ST-9 Renying.

- Second, do the wiping manipulation from BL-9 Yuzhen to GB-20 Fengchi, and the grasping manipulation, with the thumb and index finger of the right hand, toward the spinal process of C5. The whole process is called hook-pushing. This manipulation is exclusively used at EX-HN-5 Taiyang, so it is also called hook-pushing Tai Yang (Figure 4.7).

Key: Lift the upper arm, flex the elbow joint at the angle of about 120 degrees, and abduct the upper arm slightly; make the thumbs of two hands support the occipital region, flex the index fingers like a hook and do pressing manipulation at EX-HN-5 Taiyang; put the middle fingers on the index fingers, and slowly move index fingers along the Gallbladder Meridian in the temporal region towards the thumb, so that the hook-pushing EX-HN-5 Taiyang is finished.

PRESSING

Place the thumb or palm on the area or acupoint to be treated, and press gradually inwards. This is called thumb-pressing (with the thumb), and palm-pressing (with the palm) (Figure 4.8).

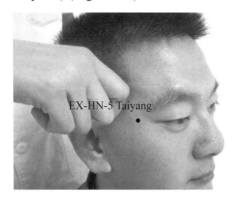

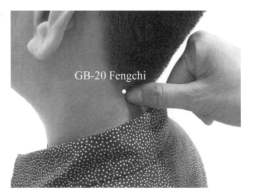

Figure 4.7 Hook-pushing (one-finger-pushing manipulation)

Figure 4.8 Pressing (one-finger-pushing manipulation)

Key: The direction of pressure should be vertical, and the strength should be increased gradually (stable and consistent), or rhythmically. In *thumb-pressing*, the thumb should be straight, using the flank to administer pressure, and the other four fingers are stretched as support. In *palm-pressing*, extend the elbow joint, sink the upper arm naturally, and do the manipulation with one hand, or overlap hands, using the heel of the hand, the thenar eminence, or the whole palm to apply pressure.

TWISTING

Hold a part of body, such as the two sides of the waist, or sternal ribs, with two palms (including thumb flanks), and twist quickly, alternately in both directions (Figure 4.9).

Key: Keep the elbow joint extended to an angle between 150 and 160 degrees, and apply the twisting movement, about 120–160 times per minute.

KNEADING

Place the thenar eminence, heel of the hand, or flank of the thumb on the area or acupoint to be treated, and do gentle, circular kneading so as to move the subcutaneous tissues. This is called heel-of-the-hand kneading (or thumb kneading) (Figure 4.10).

Key: Use the thenar eminence or heel of the hand as the point of contact, relax the wrist, and do the gentle, circular manipulation with the wrist joint and upper arm. The force should be gentle, and the frequency about 120–180 times per minute.

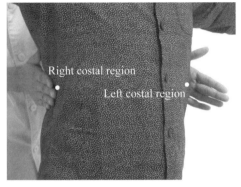 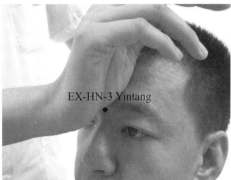

Finger 4.9 Twisting (one-finger-pushing manipulation)	*Figure 4.10 Kneading (one-finger-pushing manipulation)*

Section III Rolling Manipulation

Summary

Rolling manipulation is a clinical procedure for treating disease and injury. There are few variants of this manipulation, but it is very highly skilled. The primary manipulation is rolling and kneading, with pressing, grasping, twisting, and hold-twisting as adjunct manipulations. Rolling manipulation was developed from the ancient tradition of one-finger-pushing and also incorporates the strong points of other schools, while remaining distinct from them.

According to the theory of rolling manipulation, the pathogenesis of migraine is closely related to mental disturbance, so the treatment is mainly concerned with calming the mind, in accordance with the theory that the yang-channels from every part of the whole body converge in the neck and nape as the sole pathway along which the yang supply must flow. In case of problems in this pathway, migraine occurs; so in the process of treatment, more manipulations are applied to the neck and nape in order to clear the flow and relieve the pain.

This manipulation is applied on large areas such as the neck and nape, the upper arm, and so on. Sometimes several channel points are used, but no special acupoints. We will highlight and describe the specific manipulations in the following section.

Treatment

Therapeutic principle: Calming and tranquilizing the mind, dredging collaterals and relieving pain.

Manipulations: Rolling, kneading, pressing, and grasping.

Area: Head and face, neck and nape, shoulder.

Method: The patient sits, with eyes closed. The practitioner stands on the anterolateral side of the patient. One hand holds the occipital region, and the lateral side of thumb of the other hand kneads along five lines on the patient's head and face:

- the frontal region, from EX-HN-3 Yintang to DU-23 Shangxing

- the frontal region, from EX-HN-3 Yintang to EX-HN-5 Taiyang

- the bridge arch (sternocleidomastoid part)

- the region around the orbit (Figure 4.11)

- the temporal region, from ST-8 Touwei to EX-HN-5 Taiyang to ST-6 Jiache (Figure 4.12).

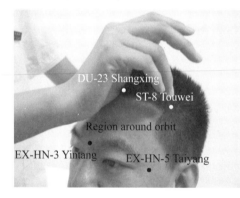 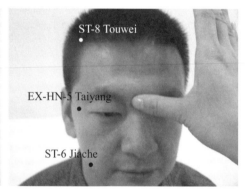

Figure 4.11 Rolling manipulation on the face and the head

Figure 4.12 Rolling manipulation on the temple

Then extend the fingers to grasp the head, with the middle finger on the Governor Channel and the other fingers on the Bladder Meridian and Gallbladder Meridian, and repeat the grasping manipulation from the frontal to occipital region (Figure 4.13). After that, do the rolling manipulation on the neck and nape with one hand, pressing the other hand against the head, so that the head and neck move passively in conjunction with the rolling manipulation. In the process of rolling:

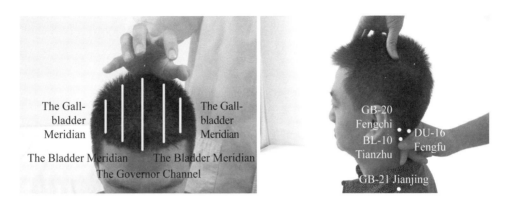

Figure 4.13 Rolling manipulation on the top of the head

Figure 4.14 Rolling manipulation on the neck and shoulder

- press GB-20 Fengchi, DU-16 Fengfu, and BL-10 Tianzhu
- grasp the muscles of the nape
- grasp GB-21 Jianjing (Figure 4.14), SJ-5 Waiguan, and LI-4 Hegu
- press GB-34 Yanglingquan, LR-3 Taichong
- and finally knead with outer flank of the thumb on the surface projection of the sympathetic trunk in the anterior region of the neck and carotid artery (Figure 4.15).

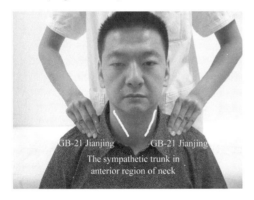

Figure 4.15 Rolling manipulation on the front of the neck

Duration of treatment: 30 minutes for a complete treatment, once a day; 20 times forms a course of treatment.

Key points

ROLLING

Place the part of the palm nearest to the little finger on the area to be treated, flex the metacarpophalangeal joint slightly, and move that part of palm continuously to-and-fro by flexing and extending the wrist joint to the maximum extent (Figure 4.16).

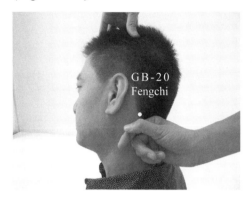

Figure 4.16 Rolling (rolling manipulation)

Key: Relax and drop the shoulder; flex the elbow joint without raising it high; keep the elbow 15cm away from your body; the fingers should be bent naturally, neither overflexed nor overextended. The range of wrist extension should be large, and more than half of the back of hand should remain in contact with the treatment area. The upper arm and forearm should be completely relaxed. Pressure should be exerted though the area near the little finger of the palm, which remains in close contact with the treatment area. There should be no moving, scrubbing, over-pressing, or bouncing; the force should be even, the movement coordinated, and the rhythm regular (never alternating between mild and strong).

KNEADING

Kneading manipulation is divided into kneading with the thenar and kneading with the outer flank of the thumb. For the former, extend the palm, flex the center of the palm slightly, place the thenar on the area to be treated, and apply helical manipulation. For the latter, place the part of the thumb between the metacarpophalangeal joint and the thumb tip on the treatment area, and make the outer flank of thumb do the up-and-down movement gently by swinging the wrist up and down (Figure 4.11).

Key: Drop the shoulder instead of lifting it, flex the elbow joint and keep it 15cm away from you, and separate the fingers a little. In thenar kneading, the facies palmaris should be flat; in the kneading with the outer flank of the thumb, the facies palmaris should be slightly tilted, and the fingers should be bent naturally, neither overflexed nor overextended. The extent of up–down or left–right motion of the wrist should be firm (not too strong or too loose), and the force should be gentle, even, and rhythmical, never alternately gentle and strong.

PRESSING

Press the area with the flank of the thumb, and apply the helical pressing and kneading manipulations to the subcutaneous level, muscles, tendons, and channels (Figure 4.17).

Key: Extend the thumb, position if accurately, and increase power gradually.

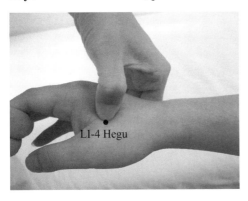

LI-4 Hegu

Figure 4.17 Pressing (rolling manipulation)

GRASPING

Hold the skin, muscles, tendons, and channels between the thumb and the other fingers, grasp slowly, then relax. Continue to grasp and relax alternately (Figure 4.15).

Section IV Manipulation According to Syndrome Differentiation

Summary

Syndrome differentiation is an aspect of Tuina manipulation based on the theory of visceral syndrome differentiation in Traditional Chinese Medicine.

In treating migraine, point selection is based on visceral syndrome differentiation as follows:

Signs of *liver yang headache* are the syndromes of:

- headache and distension

- vexation and irritability

- red eye and bitter taste in mouth

- flushed complexion and thirst in mouth

- red tongue with yellow coating

- wiry pulse or wiry-rapid pulse.

Signs of *kidney deficiency headache* are the syndromes of:

- headache and fear of cold
- cold in the limbs
- pale complexion and tongue
- deep and thready pulse.

Signs of *qi and blood deficiency headache* are the syndromes of:

- dull headache
- hypomnesia, dizziness, palpitations, and hard breath
- fatigue in limbs, which is worse after work
- lack of appetite
- pale or shallow yellow complexion, pale lips
- pale tongue with thin, white coating
- deep, thready, and weak pulse.

Signs of *poor circulation headace* are the syndromes of:

- stabbing, long-lasting, and fixed heahache
- purple and dark tongue with static-blood spots
- thready and unsmooth pulse, or wiry and slippery pulse.

Signs of *phlegm turbidity headache* are the syndromes of:

- headache as if the head were wrapped
- chest distress
- vomiting and nauseating phlegm and fluid retention
- bland taste in mouth and anorexia
- enlarged tongue with white, greasy coating or thin, white coating.

First, determine the aetiology of all syndromes (e.g. ascendant hyperactivity of liver yang; kidney qi deficiency; qi and blood deficiency; turbid phlegm obstruction stasis in channels and collaterals); then select the relevant channel points or special effective points, and carry out manipulations to treat the disease.

Treatment

Therapeutic principle: Dispelling wind and tranquilizing the mind, soothing the liver, and promoting bile secretion.

Manipulations: Pressing, kneading, one-finger-pushing manipulation, dispersing, and twisting.

Acupoints: EX-HN-5 Taiyang, ST-8 Touwei, SJ-20 Jiaosun, GB-8 Shuaigu, GB-15 Toulinqi, GB-20 Fengchi, LR-14 Qimen, GB-24 Riyue, GB-25 Jingmen.

Methods: The patient sits upright. The practitioner applies the one-finger-pushing manipulation on the area around the Gallbladder Meridian on the head for two minutes, and then kneads EX-HN-5 Taiyang, ST-8 Touwei, SJ-20 Jiaosun, GB-8 Shuaigu, GB-15 Toulinqi for one minute each. Then press the Gallbladder Meridian on the affected side with the flank of thumb, ten times. Next perform dispersing (see page 151) from the anterior superior side to the posterior inferior side of the Gallbladder Meridian, 10–20 times. After that do the manipulation on the costarum muscles in the back (Figure 4.18). Keeping the patient in the same position, knead LR-14 Qimen, GB-24 Riyue, GB-25 Jingmen for one minute per acupoint with the thumb (Figure 4.19), then press the ribs for 5–8 times with thumb, and knead and twist the lateral thorax with two hands until the skin warms up (Figure 4.20).

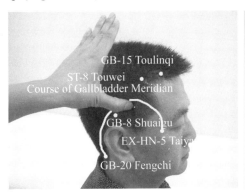

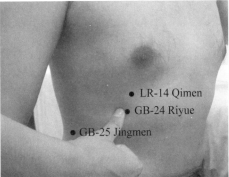

Figure 4.18 Syndrome differentiation: manipulation on the temple

Figure 4.19 Syndrome differentiation: pressing on the costal regions

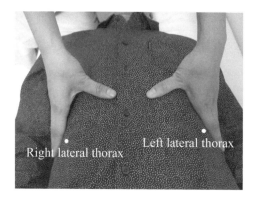

Figure 4.20 Manipulation on the costal regions (syndrome differentiation manipulation)

- **Blazing of liver-fire gallbladder:** Knead LR-3 Taichong, GB-40 Qiuxu, SJ-6 Zhigou, SJ-5 Waiguan for one minute per acupoint (Figure 4.21).

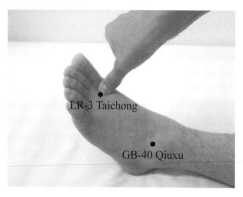

Figure 4.21 Treating blazing of liver-fire gallbladder (syndrome differentiation manipulation)

- **Liver-gallbladder dampness and heat:** Knead LR-3 Taichong, GB-34 Yanglingquan, SP-9 Yinlingquan, ST-36 Zusanli with the thumb for one minute per acupoint; knead the Gallbladder Meridian of the affected side with the thenar (Figure 4.22).

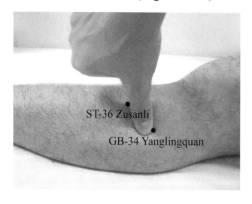

Figure 4.22 Treating liver-gallbladder dampness and heat (syndrome differentiation manipulation)

- **Wind-cold congealing and stagnation:** Knead BL-12 Fengmen and BL-13 Feishu with the thumb for one minute per acupoint; scrub BL-12 Fengmen, BL-13 Feishu until the skin warms up; press and knead GB-20 Fengchi, LI-4 Hegu for one minute per acupoint; grasp GB-20 Fengchi and the muscles of the nape for two minutes; grasp GB-21 Jianjing on both sides for one minute (Figure 4.23).

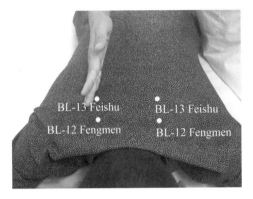

Figure 4.23 Treating wind-cold congealing and stagnation (syndrome differentiation manipulation)

- **Obstruction of meridians and collaterals:** Press and knead along the impacted course of the Gallbladder Meridian for two minutes; scrub EX-HN-5 Taiyang in the impacted part to produce heat sensation (Figure 4.24).

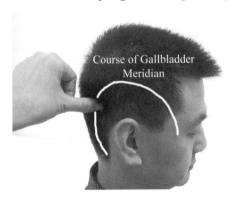

Figure 4.24 Obstruction of meridians and collaterals (syndrome differentiation manipulation)

- **Duration of treatment:** A treatment is 30 minutes, once a day, with 20 times forms a course of treatment.

Key points

PRESSING

Place the finger or palm on the area or acupoint and press gradually inwards, which is called pressing. It is called finger-pressing with the use of the finger, and palm-pressing with the use of the palm (Figure 4.21).

Key: The direction of pressing should be vertical, and the power should be from gentle to heavy, stable and constant, or rhythmical. In the process of finger-pressing, the thumb should be extended, with pressure exerted through the flank, and the other four fingers stretched as a support. In the process of palm-pressing, extend the elbow joint, drop the upper arm naturally, and either do the manipulation with one hand, or overlap the hands and exert pressure through the heel of the hand, thenar eminence, or whole palm.

KNEADING

Kneading manipulation is divided into kneading with the thenar and kneading with the outer flank of the thumb. For thenar kneading, extend the palm, flex the center of the palm a little, place the thenar on the treatment area and do the helical manipulation. For kneading with the outer flank of the thumb, place the part of the thumb between the metacarpophalangeal joint and the tip of the thumb on the treatment area, and make the outer flank of the thumb move gently up and down by swinging the wrist up and down (Figure 4.25).

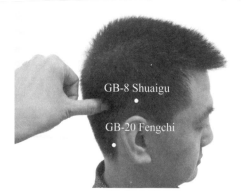

GB-8 Shuaigu

GB-20 Fengchi

Figure 4.25 Kneading (syndrome differentiation manipulation)

Key: Drop the shoulder, do not lift it; flex the shoulder joint; stand 15cm away from the patient, and separate the fingers a little. If the thenar kneading is applied, the facies palmaris should be flat; if kneading is applied with the outer flank of the thumb, the facies palmaris should be slightly tilted, and the fingers should be bent naturally, neither overflexed nor overextended. The extent of up–down or left–right motion of the wrist should be firm (not too strong or too loose), and the power should be gentle, even and rhythmical, never alternately gentle and strong.

PUSHING

Place the flank of the thumb, the facies palmaris, elbow tip, or other part of body firmly on the treatment area, acupoint, or channels, and carry out the unidirectional pushing manipulation along a straight line or curve (pushing). Finger-pushing and palm-pushing are usually applied to treat migraine (Figure 4.20):

- **Finger-pushing:** Place the flank of the thumb on the treatment area, supported by the other four separated fingers, and push forwards in the direction of the channel of the muscle. In the process of this manipulation, some gentle pressing and kneading can be applied on any particular acupoint or significant area.

- **Palm-pushing:** Place the facies palmaris tightly over the treatment area or acupoint, and push in the chosen direction with the heel of the hand. If more pressure is needed, place the palm of one hand on top of the other, and push forwards slowly.

TWISTING

Hold a part of body, such as both sides of the waist or a sternal rib, between both palms (including the flanks), and twist rapidly in opposite directions (Figure 4.26).

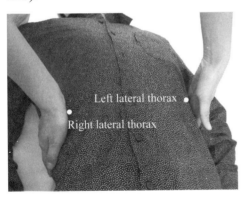

Figure 4.26 Twisting (syndrome differentiation manipulation)

Key: Keep the elbow joint open, flexed at an angle between 150 and 160 degrees; the twisting movement should be in the frequency of about 120–160 per minute.

DISPERSING

Push from EX-HN-5 Taiyang, ST-8 Touwei, and the mastoid to GB-20 Fengchi with the pads of the thumb and four fingers. Rub repeatedly over the temporal region (Figure 4.27).

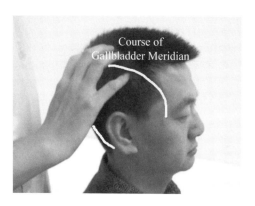

Figure 4.27 Dispersing (syndrome differentiation manipulation)

Key: One hand holds the patient's head, the thumb of the other hand is extended. Place the radial flank of the thumb at the hairline on the frontal bone, with the other four fingers (closed and slightly flexed) on the bony protrusion behind the ear and the index finger parallel to the top of the ear. Position the radial flank of the thumb and the four fingertips, and then carry out a rapid, uni-directional pushing manipulation on the temporal region. The thumb manipulates the area between the hairline of the frontal bone to the top of the ear, and the other four fingers manipulate the area from the back of the ear to the mastoid process.

PUSHING YIZHICHAN

Place the finger tip, the flank, and the tip of radialis of the thumb on the channel points or region, relax the shoulder and elbow joints, and exert a constant force on channels, points, or region by continually swinging the wrist and flexing and extending the thumb joints. This is called one-finger-pushing manipulation (Figure 4.28).

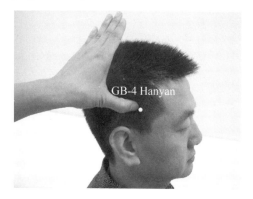

Figure 4.28 Pushing (syndrome differentiation manipulation)

Key: Relax the shoulder (relax the shoulder joint, without shrugging the shoulder); drop the elbow (relaxing the muscles of the upper limb, and dropping the elbow below the wrist); hang the wrist (hang and flex the wrist, keeping the thumb vertical so as to be able to swing the wrist left and right); position the thumb firmly (with the tip, flank, and the tip of radialis of the thumb on the treatment area, and exerting even pressure); keep the palm empty (making a hollow fist, with the four fingers away from the palm and the thumb vertical, and keeping the radialis of the middle joint of the index finger against the flank or joint of the thumb, so as to stabilize the joint activity).

Section V Manipulating Along Channels

Summary

Manipulating along channels is a combination of traditional natural therapy and modern natural therapy, and is powered by human energy. It is conducted mainly via three combinations, which encapsulate its simplicity. Meanwhile, the manipulation especially manifests such concepts in traditional medicine as "wholism" and "addressing both symptoms and root causes," showing integration in therapeutic methods, principles, and effects. Since the manipulation incorporates features of general Tuina, finger-acupuncture therapy, reflexological therapy, neuro-reflex therapy, and chiropractic therapy, it covers a wide range of clinical applications.

According to the theory of manipulations along channels, migraine is closely related to clear yang failing to ascend, and blockage of channels and collaterals in the head. Therefore, those manipulations are included which have such effects as tonifying the brain and calming the spirit; awaking the spirit and opening the orifices; dredging channels and activating collaterals; resolving spasm and relieving pain; and removing wind and activating collaterals.

There are two commonly used acupoints that are special. One is the Area of Original Spirit, which is the area surrounded by the six acupoints that include DU-17 Naohu, GB-20 Fengchi, SI-15 Jianzhongshu. The other is the Area of the Elbow Centrum, a square area located on the medial side of the upper extremities: taking cubital crease as the baseline, the area lies 2 cun above and 2 cun below the baseline.

Treatment

Therapeutic principle: Awaking the brain and calming the spirit; dredging collaterals and relieving pain.

Manipulations: Wiping, pushing, scrubbing, rolling, grasping, channel rubbing, tapping.

Methods: The treatment methods are outlined in the sections below.

WIPING THE EYEBROWS

The patient is seated, facing, and the therapist stands, facing the patient. Wipe with the thumbs from EX-HN-3 Yintang, along the eyebrows to EX-HN-5 Taiyang, 15–30 times (Figure 4.29).

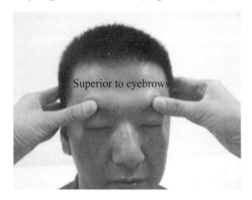

Figure 4.29 Wiping the eyebrows (manipulation along channels)

PUSHING THE TEMPLES THREE TIMES

Maintaing the same position, push with the ring fingers from the beginning of the Taiyang Meridian along the channel, following a line above the ears, as far as GB-20 Fengchi on the nape. Meanwhile, push with the thumbs, from the hairline at the corners of the forehead down to the temples, and then push from ST-8 Touwei and EX-HN-3 Yintang to GB-20 Fengchi. Each track should be covered 15–30 times (Figure 4.30).

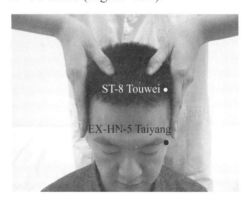

Figure 4.30 Pushing the temples three times (manipulation along channels)

RUBBING WITH SWORD-SHAPED FINGERS

The patient remains sitting. Stand behind the patient, and bring the middle finger and the ring finger together to make them look like a sword, on both hands. Lay the pads of the fingers on GB-8 Shuaigu, and the thumbs at the back of the head, and push continuously back and forth laterally, about 15–30 times (Figure 4.31).

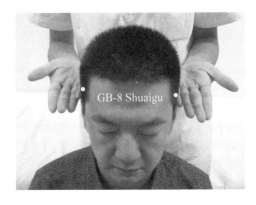

Figure 4.31 Rubbing with sword-shaped fingers (manipulations along channels)

POINT-TAPPING

Maintain the same position. Bend the fingers to make them look like a tiger-paw, on both hands. Then tap from the anterior hairline to the occiput, 10–15 times (Figure 4.32).

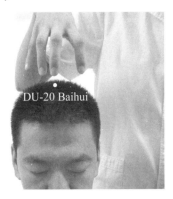

Figure 4.32 Point-tapping (manipulations along channels)

GRASPING AND KNEADING THE SHOULDERS AND NECK

Stay in the same position. Grasp GB-20 Fengchi. Grasp and knead the patient's shoulders and neck. After that, push the Area of Original Spirit for several minutes (Figure 4.33).

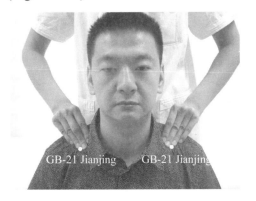

Figure 4.33 Grasping and kneading the shoulders and neck (manipulations along channels)

TAPPING THE ELBOW ALONG THE CHANNELS

The patient is seated. The physician faces the patient, on the side that is to be treated. Lift the patient's arm with one hand. Loosely grasp the shoulder with the thumb, pushing quite hard with the other hand, and rub along the channels and collaterals of the upper arm, about ten times. Then roll the Area of the Elbow Centrum, about 50 times. Use the same hand to form a hollow fist, half-closed and with half-bent fingers. Tap the Area of the Elbow Centrum about 15–30 times (Figure 4.34).

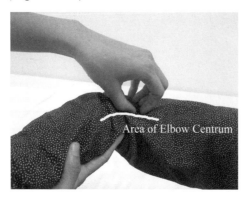

Figure 4.34 Tapping the elbow along the channels (manipulations along channels)

FINGER-PUSHING CHANNELS AND COLLATERALS

Stay in the same position. Free the hand holding the patient's upper arm and place it on the patient's palm. Place the pad of the thumb of the treating hand on the medial side of the second metacarpal. Push with the thumb repeatedly, about 100 times (Figure 4.35).

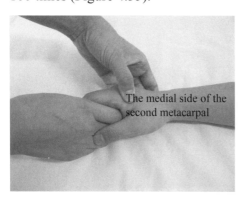

Figure 4.35 Finger-pushing channels and collaterals (manipulations along channels)

Key points

WIPING

With one or both hands, wipe back and forth over the target area, slowly and smoothly with the pad of the thumb (Figure 4.29).

PUSHING

With one or both hands: use the thumbs, or bring the index finger and the middle, or the index finger and the ring finger together and apply the pads of the thumbs or fingers to the target area; push along the channels and collaterals repeatedly. Finger pushing is one of two types of pushing. Only this one is introduced here, as it is applied in migraine treatment (Figure 4.30).

SCRUBBING

Apply finger pads or the palms to the target area, and push repeadedly or scrub along the channels and collaterals (Figure 4.31).

TAPPING

With one or both hands, bend the fingers, and let the elbow and wrist lead the finger tips to tap the target area (Figure 4.32).

GRASPING

With one or both hands, form a clamp with the thumb and four fingers, then grasp and knead the target area (Figure 4.33).

PRESSING ALONG CHANNELS

Apply pads of the thumb or the palms to the target area, and rub and knead along the channels and collaterals in a straight line or in circles (Figure 4.34).

ROLLING

Make a hollow fist, then apply back of the hand to the target area, and roll it back and forth.

Section VI Acupressure

Summary

Acupressure therapy is a mode of treatment in which the physician presses the patient's acupoints with one or both hands. The therapy introduced here originated from Southern Fujian culture, developed over years of civil spreading and sorted by later generations.

The therapy is based on the theory that migraine occurs when the body lacks yang qi and loses protection against external pathogens, or else incubates internal pathogens due to the failure of yang qi to push. As a result, external or internal pathogens block local channels and collaterals, leading to blockage of channel qi, and pain. Special acupoints, which were considered capable of stimulating yang qi and dredging channels and collaterals in the head, were selected for stimulation, with the aim of activating yang and collaterals, eliminating pathogens, and relieving pain.

Acupoint-taking in this therapy differs from that in traditional acupuncture, because it is based on conclusions drawn from a large body of clinical cases carrying positive reaction points and injury parts. In this sense, it is to some extent related to, but not completely the same as, Ashi points. Acupoints that are usually applied in this therapy to migraine treatment are as follows.

- **Cranial point:** A depression on the lower rim of the occipital tuberosity (point-press upwards).

- **Temporal point:** A depression 1 cun behind the external canthus (point-press).

- **Vertebral point:** 0.5cm away from the line between the C7 and T1 vertebrae (point-press or grasp the outward side).

- **Scuttle point:** At the midpoint of the line between the earlobe and the occipital tuberosity (point-press or grasp inwards and upwards).

- **Paraoccipital point:** 1.5cm away from the line between C1 and C7 (point-press perpendicularly, or pluck).

- **Medial Eye-brow point:** As the medial point of the superciliary arch (point-press upwards).

- **Yangming point:** At the midpoint of the forehead, 0.5cm above the anterior hairline (point-press perpendicularly).

- **Brain Orifice point:** 1.5cm above the Scuttle point (thumb-press or grasp).

- **Super-auricular point:** Fold the ear forward; 1 cun above the ear tip (point-push backwards).

- **Eighteenth Channel:** 0.5cm away from the line between C7 and L5 (point-press or pluck outwards).

Treatment

Therapeutic principle: Dredging yang and activate collaterals, eliminating pathogen, and relieving pain.

Manipulations: Point-pressing, point-pushing, point-plucking, grasping.

Therapeutic areas: Cranial point, Temporal point, Vertebral point, Scuttle point, Paraoccipital point, Medial Eye-brow point, Yangming point, Brain Orifice point, Super-auricular point, Eighteenth Channel.

Methods: Forcefully grasp the Brain Orifice point; point-press the Cranial point and the Scuttle point; press-push and press-pluck the Paraoccipital point; point-press the Vertebral point (Figure 4.36). Point-push the Eighteenth Channel (Figure 4.37); point-press the Medial Eye-brow point; push upwards from the Medial Eye-brow point to the Yangming point; point-press the Yangming point (Figure 4.38). Point-press the Temporal point and the Super-auricular point (Figure 4.39).

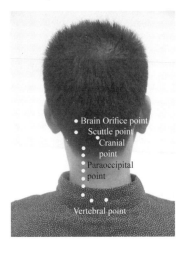

Figure 4.36 Point selection for acupoint-pressing therapy on the head and neck

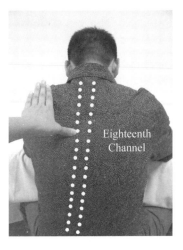

Figure 4.37 Point selection for acupoint-pressing therapy on the back

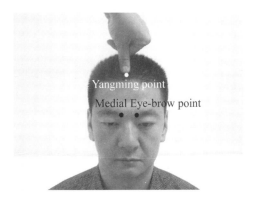

Figure 4.38 Point selection for acupoint pressing therapy on the face

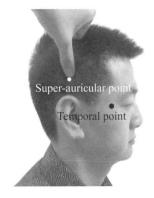

Figure 4.39 Point selection for acupoint pressing therapy on the temple

Duration of treatment: Press each point for 3–5 minutes, for a maximum of 30 minutes in total, once a day, ten times forms a course of treatment.

Key points

POINT-PRESSING

Press perpendicularly downwards onto the point with the pad or tip of the thumb, index finger, or middle finger. Make spiral movements on the points while pressing (Figure 4.39).

Key: Press with the finger pad or thumb, and make spiral movements on the points while pressing. Press perpendicularly downwards with the forearm and wrist, gradually increasing the force. Press the finger tips or pads against the body surface, and do not scrub the surface while making spiral movements.

POINT-PUSHING

Press the point with the pad of the thumb and push slowly (Figure 4.37).

Key: Press with the pad of finger, and push slowly. The upper arm, forearm, and wrist together move the pad of the thumb. Otherwise, use major thenar eminence to move the pad of the thumb transversely. Stay close to the body surface, and move steadily, evenly, and slowly in the chosen direction.

POINT-PLUCKING

Pluck the tendon on the point with the pad or tip of the thumb, back and forth (Figure 4.40).

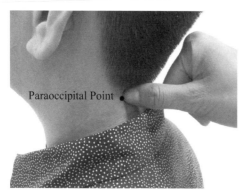

Paraoccipital Point

Figure 4.40 Point-pushing (acupoint pressing therapy)

Key: Relax the shoulders and wrist. Separate the thumb from the other fingers. Fix the four fingers. Place pad or tip of the thumb on the tendon, or press in on one side of the tendon. Fix the thumb on the tendon, then pluck, applying an even force, speed, and stimulus.

GRASPING

Clamp the target area between the thumb and the other four fingers symmetrically. Slowly lift, and release. Repeat several times (Figure 4.41).

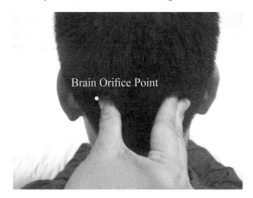

Brain Orifice Point

Figure 4.41 Grasping (acupoint pressing therapy)

Section VII Finger-Pressing Acupoints of the Chest

Summary

Finger-pressing on the acupoints of the chest is based on theories concerning the surface of the body and internal organs. Manipulations are applied to stimulate the surface of the chest bones and neighbouring sensitive points, to treat disease. The theory mainly originates from Western medicine, on the basis that the sensory nerve fibers of a particular internal organ, together with the sensory nerve fibers of related skin, muscles, and bones, all link into the same spinal segment. Therefore, when an internal organ is dysfunctional, reactive pain or pressure points are seen in the related areas on the surface of the body. These pain or pressure points are the ones that need to be stimulated by finger-pressing; they are also called chest acupoints.

The theory of chest acupoints states that migraine occurs when the neural segments that control sense and movement of the head fail to function normally, or when other Zang-Fu organs or tissues controlled by the same segment malfunction. Therefore, during treatment, stimulation of other parts of the same neural segment can achieve beneficial results. From a Traditional Chinese Medicine perspective, this theory is in agreement with one-finger-pushing manipulation theory with regard to migraine. They both hold that migraine is caused by ascendant hyperactivity of liver yang, which disturbs mental processes.

Since chest acupoint therapy has its own unique theory, its point-taking is different from that of traditional treatment. Commonly used acupoints in migraine treatment include the following:

- **Supraclavicular 2:** One finger-breadth medial to the midpoint of the supraclavicular brim, on the inner side of the clavicle. There are two ways of taking points. One is to place the thumb in the supraclavicular fossae and move the thumbs gently: the point is where the physician's thumb feels something like a thin rope rolling inside, while the patient feels distending pain on the temporal side. The other is to press the thumbs against the supraclavicular fossae, backwards and downwards. The point is identifiable by the patient's feeling of numbness and distension in the scapula and the ulnar side of the arm.

- **Supraspinatus 1:** At the corner of the spine of the scapula.

Finger-pressing on chest acupoints, which is characterized by softness and deepness, strength contained inside, and penetration into acupoints, can be described as "pressing," "sliding," "vibrating," and "striking." "Pressing" and "sliding" comprise three different aims respectively: to meet the needs of different diseases, therapeutic areas, and patients. In migraine treatment, the manipulations applied are mainly circling thumb pressure and sliding with the thumbs. These procedures are described on the following page.

Treatment

Therapeutic principle: Tonifying the kidneys and pacifying the liver, tranquilizing counterflow, and relieving pain.

Manipulations: Circular finger pressure, sliding the fingers.

Therapeutic points: Supraclavicular 2, supraspinatus 1.

Methods: Slide the thumb over supraclavicular 2 (Figure 4.42) and supraspinatus 1 (Figure 4.43), and then perform circling thumb pressure on pressure points on the head.

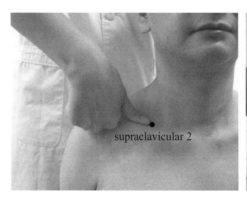
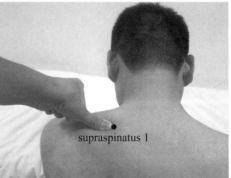

Figure 4.42 Point-selection
for supraclavicular 2

Figure 4.43 Point-selection
for supraspinatus 1

Duration of treatment: Ten minutes for each point, 30 minutes for a complete treatment, once a day, ten times forms a course of treatment.

Key points

CIRCLING FINGER PRESSURE

Press the thumb against the chest acupoints. Push with the forearm and make circling movements around the chest acupoints. The range of circling should move inwards, and the circling force should be less than the downward pressure. Primarily use the circling movement and add the downward pressure last. This manipulation can assure that fingers stay with the acupoints and cover a wide range, creating a strong reaction.

SLIDING PRESSURE

Press the thumb against the chest acupoints and slide it over the rim or surface of the bones. Adjust the force of the pressure and keep it within the tolerance of the patient (Figure 4.42 and 4.43).

Section VIII Manipulation on Acupoints of the Arm

Summary

"Acupoints of the arm" means all the acupoints around the arm region. The development of manipulation on the arm acupoints was inspired by Tuina for children and ear points. Similar to the Quan Xi points, its main points are along the channels, but they are not meridian points.

The theory of manipulation on arm acupoints and the theory of Quan Xi points share some similar views about the treatment of disease. Taking the treatment of migraine as the case in point, both theories believe that stimulating specific points (arm points or Quan Xi points) that correspond to points around the head will cure the disease. In addition, the theory of manipulation on arm acupoints holds that diseases manifesting pain usually have something to do with a "sinew knot" located around the diseased area. The "sinew knot" may be either visible or invisible, and when it is not convenient to treat directly on the disease area, corresponding arm points can be worked with manipulations to reduce or eliminate the "sinew knot," so that the disease itself can be relieved or cured.

This therapy includes application of traditional acupoints, extra acupoints, and some specific acupoints. Points used in the treatment of migraine are mainly along the channel, and include the three following.

- **Bi Tai Yang:** LI-15 Jianyu above the deltoid, between the acromion and the humerus, below the anterior of the hollow formed by sideways movement of the arm.

- **Bi Feng Fu:** Medial of LI-14 Binao, 7 cun above LI-11 Quchi, along the posterior edge of deltoid as far as the hollow. It is the point corresponding to the C1 vertebra.

- **Bi Yin Tang:** Below the anterior of the shoulder protuberance, two finger-breadths from the axilla crease, at the midpoint of the biceps brachii tendon.

Treatment

Therapeutic principle: Relaxing the sinews and relieving pain.

Manipulations: Kneading, point-pressing, pressing.

Therapeutic areas: Bi Tai Yang, Bi Feng Fu, Bi Yin Tang, LI-11 Quchi, EX-HN-5 Taiyang, PC-7 Daling, TE-14 Jianliao, TE-13 Naohui.

Methods: Mainly stimulate Bi Tai Yang and LI-11 Quchi. Use one thumb to knead and point-press Bi Tai Yang on the affected side (Figure 4.44); meanwhile use the other thumb to knead and point-press LI-11 Quchi (Figure 4.45). The two hands can work alternately. During treatment, observe the condition of abnormal tissues carefully, including size and stiffness. Migraine will be relieved if the abnormal tissues become softer, smaller, or are even eliminated after a period of manipulation. Other points are treated with kneading, point-pressing, and pressing from above to below (Figure 4.46).

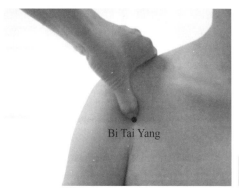

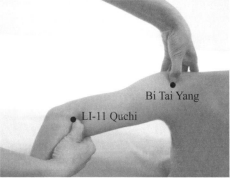

Figure 4.44 Manipulation on arm acupoints (upper arm)

Figure 4.45 Manipulation on arm acupoints (elbow)

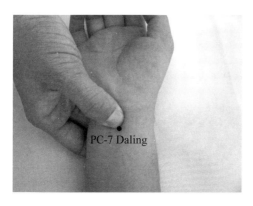

PC-7 Daling

*Figure 4.46 Method of manipulation
on arm acupoints (forearm)*

Duration of treatment: Five to ten minutes for each point, 30 minutes for a complete treatment, once a day, ten times forms a course of treatment.

Key points

KNEADING

Apply some strength on the area or acupoints. Use the pad of the thumb to do spiral movements softly and gently, and also to transmit movement into the subcutaneous tissue (Figure 4.45).

POINT-PRESSING

Use the tip or flexed second knuckle of the thumb to point-press the area, and knead and press down into deeper tissues (Figure 4.46).

Key: When using the tip of the thumb to press points, a hollow fist is required and the strength of pressure is generated mainly from the forearm and wrist. When using the knuckle, the fist, by contrast, should be clenched, and the strength of pressure is again generated from the forearm and wrist. Point-pressing should be applied tightly against body surface, and strength should be gradually increased, to reach down into deeper layers under the surface.

PRESSING

Use the thumbs to apply force on the area or acupoints, and gradually increase it to go deeper (Figure 4.47).

Key: The direction of pressing should be vertical, the strength should be gradually increased, and the pressure should be stable and constant or rhythmical. When using the thumb for pressing, it is important to keep it straight, applying force through the pad of the thumb, and stretching the four fingers to support it.

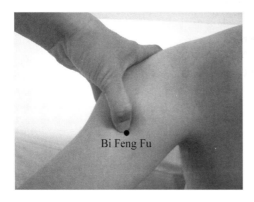

Bi Feng Fu

Figure 4.47 Kneading (manipulation on arm acupoints)

Section IX Self-Tuina

Summary

Self-Tuina is massage or Tuina practised on oneself to prevent and treat disease. As a traditional method of health care, it belongs to the category of ancient conduction, and has been a source of great benefit. This therapy has a long history, and a wide repertoire of techniques. Characteristic of it is the integration of "thought," "qi," and "form." For certain chronic diseases, it has the advantage that treatment can be given regardless of time and place.

As a kind of chronic disease, migraine can be treated by self-Tuina. Self-Tuina assists prevention on a daily basis, and brings relief in cases of onset. We now introduce two easy procedures for self-Tuina.

Treatment

The key areas for stimulation when treating migraine with self-Tuina are on the head and face. Since most cases suffer discomfort, distension, and pain in the eyes before or during migraine attacks, you should cover your eyes while doing self-Tuina.

WIPING THE HEAD

Keep the index finger, middle finger, and ring finger close together, and perform Tuina along the following three paths in sequence.

1. Wipe from EX-HN-3 Yintang via DU-23 Shangxing and over the top of head to DU-14 Dazhui, ten times (Figure 4.48).

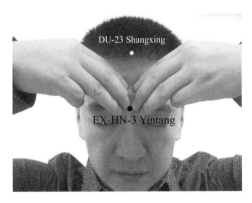

Figure 4.48 Point-pressing (manipulation on arm acupoints)

2. Wipe from the temples and behind the ears to GB-21 Jianjing, ten times (Figure 4.49).

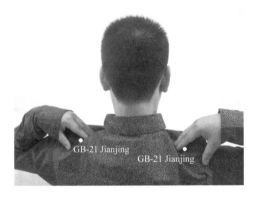

Figure 4.49 Pressing (manipulation on arm acupoints)

3. Work downwards from EX-HN-5 Taiyang and in front of the ears, to ST-9 Renying, ten times (Figure 4.50).

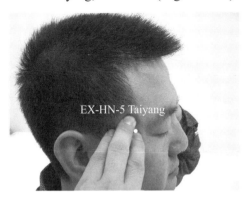

Figure 4.50 Wiping the head (self-Tuina)

RUBBING THE EYES

Softly close the eyes. Gently, with the pads of the fingers, rub the eyes from the medial side to the lateral side, ten times. Open the eyes and look straight ahead.

Rotate the eyeballs alternately clockwise and anti-clockwise, five times (Figure 4.51).

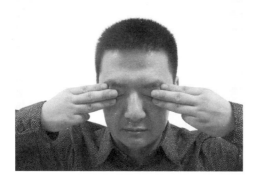

Figure 4.51 Rubbing the eyes (self-Tuina)

Key points

Take care when rubbing the eyes. Make sure the rubbing is soft and gentle and do not continue for too long. Stop when the eyes feel warm.

Note: This method is only applicable to mild migraine, or for temporary relief of symptoms.

Chapter 5

Case Studies

Experienced acupoint BL-67 Zhiyin

Patient Wang is a 50-year-old man. His first consultation is on 15 April 2007.

The patient has had migraine on the right side for about ten years. Onset has become increasingly frequent over the past year. There are between three and six attacks of headache each month. Now the amount of sedative and anaesthetic medication needed is two or three times more than it originally was. However, the headache is still not relieved. The patient now has to take strong sedative and pain-relieving medication to ease the pain every one to two hours. He sleeps badly at night, and feels drowsy and dull by day. The headache occurs or worsens following insomnia. Several CT and MRI scans on the head have revealed no space-occupying lesion. Ophthalmologic and ENT examinations are also normal.

The patient's symptoms are: headache on the right side; the pain radiating to the right side of the forehead; facial pain; dizziness; slightly closed eyes; photophobia; low voice; red tongue with yellow coating; wiry, tight pulse.

Diagnosis: Migraine.

Acupoints: BL-67 Zhiyin.

Manipulation: Insert 1 cun filiform needle. The needle is retained for 30 minutes. Squeeze for several drops of blood on withdrawing the needle.

Effect: Pain in the right side of the head is relieved after acupuncture treatment. The headache is relieved after 12 treatments. There is no recurrence during follow-up.

Notes: One of the important acupoint selection principles is to choose acupoints along the meridian pathway. BL-67 Zhiyin belongs to the Bladder Meridian. The Bladder Meridian pathway originates at the inner canthus and runs upward to the apex of the head. One branch separates from the apex and runs superior to the ear. Another branch enters into the brain from the apex of the head, and then exits from the neck (*Spiritual Pivot, Discussion on Meridians*). So the Bladder Meridian passes through the forehead, the apex, back, and side of the head.

The meridian branch that separates from the apex and runs superior to the ear treats pain on the side of the head.

BL-67 Zhiyin, the most yin acupoint, is used to treat disease of the head, which is the place of the most yang, and the method of using BL-67 Zhiyin to treat headache is recorded in ancient literature. In recent clinical practice, Professor Wei Jia also reports thte positive therapeutic effect of using BL-67 Zhiyin to treat migraine. Therefore, BL-67 Zhiyin is an effective acupoint for treating migraine.

Single acupoint GB-20 Fengchi

Patient Zhang is an 18-year-old girl. Her first consultation is on 24 June 2005.

The patient has had migraine on the left side for two years: the pain began of late due to stress while preparing for an examination. Severe, paroxysmal pain occurs several times a day on the left side of the head. The pain radiates to the auricular and occipital regions. The severe pain causes nausea, vomiting, poor concentration, restlessness, drowsiness, and stress. No abnormality was shown in brain CT. Oral administration of pain-relieving drugs is not effective. The patient requested acupuncture treatment.

Diagnosis: Migraine.

Acupoints: GB-20 Fengchi (left side).

Manipulation: The patient sits, with her head tilted to one side. Disinfect around the acupoints. Insert a 1.5 cun (size 28) needle into GB-20 Fengchi, with the tip of the needle aimed towards the contralateral eyeball. Manipulate the needle with strong stimulation (lifting-thrusting and twirling method) to cause numbness or the sensation of distension. Press the area below GB-20 Fengchi and continue to manipulate the needle with the right hand, so that the needling sensation spreads gradually upward to EX-HN-5 Taiyang or the apex of the head.

Effect: Migraine is obviously relieved half an hour after acupuncture treatment. The patient receives five treatments. There is no recurrence in the six-month follow-up.

Notes: The Gallbladder Meridian passes through the side of the head. GB-20 Fengchi belongs to the Gallbladder Meridian. It is an important acupoint on the head for dispersing wind, releasing exterior (the skin of the body), clearing the head, and improving vision. GB-20 Fengchi is located in between the sternocleidomastoid muscle and the trapezius muscle. The deeper muscle layer is the splenius muscle. The lesser occipital nerve also passes through this region. Acupuncture on GB-20 Fengchi is effective for relieving muscle spasm and releasing compression of blood vessels and nerves. The treatment also stimulates the lesser occipital nerve to regulate blood vessel function on the side of the head, to treat migraine.

Distal acupoint

Patient Li is a 28-year-old woman. Her first consultation is on 20 October 1993.

The patient has suffered from headache for two years. Severe headache on the right side occurs when she is tired or angry. Paroxysmal symptoms are blurred vision; paroxysmal amaurosis; pain in the orbital region, forehead, and cheek. The patient has severe headache with nausea and vomiting. The pain has become frequent and persistent over the past six months. Vascular migraine has been diagnosed by several hospitals.

The patient presents with pain on the right side of the head; copious sweating; pale complexion; pain in the face. There is no abnormality in the anterior segment and the eye ground. Intraocular pressure is normal. No abnormality is shown on brain CT. The electrocardiogram is normal. Blood pressure is 100/60 mmHg.

Diagnosis: Migraine.

Acupoints: SJ-6 Zhigou and GB-41 Zulinqi.

Manipulation: The acupoints should be located accurately. The needling depth is dependent on obtaining qi. Manipulate the needle with the lifting–thrusting, trembling method. Massage along the channel to send the needling sensation to from the arm or leg to the body.

Effect: Pain is instantly relieved after acupuncture, but recurs later. The patient receives ten treatments. No recurrence is reported during two-year follow-up.

Notes: Migraine is usually caused by heat stagnation in the Shaoyang Meridian of the head. Select SJ-6 Zhigou of the Sanjiao Meridian as the distal acupoint. If the pain is not relieved, combine it with GB-41 Zulinqi of the Gallbladder Meridian. In severe migraine cases, GB-20 Fengchi should also be combined to regulate meridian qi in the head (if the pain is not relieved by using the preceding acupoints).

Distal acupoint combined with local acupoint

Patient Fu is a 30-year-old woman. Her first consultation is on 5 November 2007.

The patient has suffered from migraine on the right side for 20 years. Frequent attacks occur during autumn and winter. The patient's medication is Naoqing tablets and Zhengtian pills. The pain lasts for about 20 days. The patient has premature menstruation, with headache before menstruation. The patient is depressed and easily loses her temper; the latest attack of headache is the result of an argument with her husband.

The patient passed out, and regained consciousness, after puncturing of DU-26 Renzhong and PC-6 Neiguan. Then she felt a heavy sensation and pain on the right side of her head, and difficulty opening her eyes. Accompanying symptoms are: blurred vision; poor memory; tiredness; restlessness; dry stools; normal appetite; red tongue with yellow coating; and wiry pulse.

Diagnosis: Migraine.

Acupoints: GB-41 Zulinqi, SJ-5 Waiguan, SJ-23 Sizhukong, GB-20 Fengchi.

Manipulation: Direct the needling sensation of GB-41 Zulinqi and SJ-5 Waiguan to the central part of the body. The needling sensation of GB-20 Fengchi should spread to the apex of the head. Penetrating needling from SJ-23 Sizhukong to GB-8 Shuaigu should cause soreness and distension on one side of the head. Wrap moxa around the handle of the needle for warming needle moxibustion.

Effect: The pain is relieved after acupuncture treatment. The heavy sensation and blurred vision disappear following treatment. The headache is cured after 20 treatments. Other symptoms are also relieved, and the patient no longer feels restlessness. The patient is encouraged to remain in a good emotional state and maintain a good balance between work and relaxation. There has been no recurrence during follow-up so far.

Notes:

- The acupoints where the eight extraordinary meridians and the 12 meridians meet are called the confluence points of the eight extraordinary meridians. These eight acupoints treat diseases of the eight extraordinary meridians as well as the 12 meridians. Dou Hanqin said in the Jin-Yuan dynasty that these acupoints are experienced points. (He learned it from a hermit.)

- SJ-5 Waiguan is connected with SJ-16 Tianyou on the shoulder via the Sanjiao Meridian, and meets the Yang Link Channel. GB-41 Zulinqi goes to the hypochondrium via the Gallbladder Meridian, and connects with the Belt Channel. These two acupoints are used to treat diseases of the outer canthus, cheek, neck, posterior of the ear, shoulder, and scapula. This is effective in treating migraine of the Shaoyang Meridian pathway.

- GB-20 Fengchi is used to dispel wind and relieve pain.

- SJ-23 Sizhukong is used to dredge meridians on the head.

- Warming needle moxibustion is used to strengthen the effect of acupuncture, warm meridians, activate blood, and relieve pain. It is effective in relieving the symptoms of severe migraine.

Hua Tuo Jiaji points

Patient Yu is a 35-year-old female office worker. Her first consultation is on 21 October 1999.

The patient has suffered from migraine on the left side for 15 years. The throbbing pain occurs when she is in a bad mood, or tired. In the beginning the pain could be reduced by a small amount of medication, but for the past year ergotamine has failed to reduce the pain. Most recently the headache started on the forehead and spread to the left side and then the entire head. It is accompanied by vomiting and poor appetite. Brain CT has ruled out the possibility of space-occupying disease.

Diagnosis: Migraine.

Acupoints: Hua Tuo Jiaji points (T5, 7, 9, 11, 14) and GB-20 Fengchi.

Manipulation: Insert 1 cun filiform needles on the Hua Tuo Jiaji points, with the tips of the needles towards the spine. Lift and thrust the needles to cause soreness and distension. The needling sensation of GB-20 Fengchi should be radiated to the apex of the head.

Effect: Treatment is given every other day. Headache is obviously relieved after ten acupuncture treatments. Fifteen acupuncture treatments are given to maintain the effect. There is not recurrence during one-year follow-up.

Notes:

- Hua Tuo Jiaji points (see page 88) are first recorded in the book of *Zhou Hou Bei Ji Fang* (*Emergency Formulas to Keep up One's Sleeve*). Hua Tuo Jiaji points are located 0.5 cun lateral to the spine, on either side of the T1 to L5 vertebral processes. These 34 acupoints are close to Back-Shu points and have a similar therapeutic effect. They are usually used to treat chronic diseases.

- Clinical practice shows that Zang-Fu disorders are represented in points on the back, which are called positive reaction points. Hua Tuo Jiaji points (T5, 7, 9, 11, 14) have the function of regulating related Zang-Fu organ function, similar to the back-Shu points of BL-15 Xinshu, BL-17 Geshu, BL-18 Ganshu, BL-20 Pishu, and BL-23 Shenshu.

- The points are used to nourish qi and blood, extinguish wind, and dredge collaterals, in order to adjust Zang-Fu organ function and expel pathogens.

- GB-20 Fengchi is used to dispel wind, improve vision, and activate meridian qi on the head to relieve headache.

Suspended moxibustion

Patient Ye is a 43-year-old man. His first consultation is in February 2003.

The patient has suffered from headache on the left side for 11 years. The pain alternates between severe and moderate. It has been severe in the past month, due to tiredness from work. The pain radiates to the left eye and affects sleep. It is accompanied by tinnitus, dizziness, numbness on the left side of the body, and retarded sensation. Appetite is normal. The tongue coating is thin and white. The pulse is thready and deep. Tender points are found near T4.

Diagnosis: Migraine.

Acupoints: DU-14 Dazhui and the point below T4.

Manipulation: Suspended moxibustion is used on DU-14 Dazhui and the point below T4. Blow the ignited end to make it burn. The moxibustion treatment is given for 25 minutes. The moxibustion sensation should spread slowly upwards to the neck and the apex of the head, and then spread to the painful areas.

Effect: The pain will be relieved when the moxibustion sensation spreads to the head. The treatment is repeated ten times, with the same moxibustion sensation. No recurrence is reported during follow-up.

Notes:

- Most cases of headache will have tender points on the Governor Channel in the thoracic region. The tender points will be found on the same side as the migraine.

- Blowing the ignited end of the moxa stick is the easiest way of making the moxibustion sensation spread to the painful area. Sometimes the sensation spreads first to the apex of the head, and then to the painful area to relieve the pain. In a few cases the sensation does not spread to the affected area, but is still effective in relieving pain.

- Besides moxibustion on the positive reaction points on the Governor Channel, direct moxibustion on DU-14 Dazhui is also effective in relieving pain. The treatment effect is also good with local acupoints, such as EX-HN-5 Taiyang, GB-20 Fengchi, EX-HN-6 Erjian.

- Moxibustion on DU-22 Xinhui is effective in treating migraine, according to the book *Classic of Nourishing Life with Acupuncture and Moxibustion* (*Zhen Jiu Zi Sheng Jing*) by Wang Zhizhong.

Ear acupuncture

Patient Wang is a 17-year-old female student. Her first consultation is on 14 August 2001.

The patient has suffered from migraine on the left side of the head for three years. The pain becomes severe due to tiredness and contact with wind-cold. It is accompanied by nausea, vomiting, and blurred vision.

The neurological examination result is normal. There is no abnormality on brain CT. The ophthalmologic examination is normal. The pain cannot be controlled by medication. The tongue is red, with thin coating. The pulse is slippery.

Diagnosis: Migraine.

Acupoints: Ear Apex, Temple, Subcortex, Sympathetic Nerve, Shenmen.

Manipulation: Press and massage the auricle of the ear to make the entire ear red. Disinfect the ear, and prick the apex of the ear for 10–20 drops of blood. Embed the needles on other points of the ear and fix them with tape. Press each point continuously.

Effect: The headache is obviously relieved after ten minutes' treatment. The pain is totally relieved after 30 minutes' treatment. The needles are embedded for two days. The frequency of onset is obviously reduced. Mild migraine occurs occasionally. The treatment is repeated seven times. There is no recurrence during the three-month follow-up.

Notes:

- In the book of *Huangdi Neijing*: *Miraculous Pivot, Discussion on Questions*, it is recorded that the ear is the gathering place of all meridians. It indicates the close relation between ear and the meridian system. Stimulating the ear acupoints is effective for dredging the entire meridian system and harmonizing qi and blood, in order to treat migraine.

- In the book of *Huangdi Neijing*: *Miraculous Pivot, Discussion on Juebing*, it is recorded that dilated blood vessels and heat cause severe headache. The treatment should be, first, bloodletting on the blood vessels, and then treatment on the Shaoyang Gallbladder Meridian of the Foot; and so bloodletting therapy is used on the apex of the ear and Helix point 6, to clear the head and improve vision.

- The temples may be selected, depending on the painful area. The forehead and occipital area can also be combined, depending on the case.

- The subcortex contains subcortex of the nerve system, cardiovascular system and digestive system. The nerve system and cardiovascular system subcortex are used to treat migraine. Sympathetic nerve can also be added in the treatment.

Plum-blossom needle

Patient Hu is a 37-year-old woman. Her first consultation is on 17 April 2008.

The patient has suffered from left-side headache with blurred vision for two years. During a pain attack, the patient cannot open her eyes. It is accompanied by throbbing pain on the left side of the head, mild nausea, poor sleep, tiredness, quick temper, and constipation. The pain occurs or becomes severe due to bad temper or tiredness. The tongue coating is thin and pale. The pulse is deep and thready. No space-occupying change is found on brain CT. The patient used to take modern medicine and Chinese medicine, with no effect. The neurological examination is normal. There is no abnormality of the heart and the lungs. Blood pressure is 110/70mmHg. Tender points are found on the neck and the superclavicular fossa. Positive reaction nodules are found lateral to vertebrae T5 to T10.

Diagnosis: Migraine.

Acupoints: Back region of the neck; area lateral to T5 to T10; lumbosacral region; temple area on the affected side; EX-HN-5 Taiyang, DU-20 Baihui, GB-20 Fengchi.

Manipulation: Tap the back of the neck and GB-20 Fengchi with a plum-blossom needle, with medium strength. Heavy tapping can be used lateral to C1 and the superclavicular fossa, to cause bleeding. Heavy tapping is also used lateral to T5 to T10, and on positive reaction points on the lumbosacral region. Mild tapping is used on the temple region, EX-HN-5 Taiyang and DU-20 Baihui of the affected side, to cause redness on the local area.

Effect: The pain is relieved after one treatment. The onset of headache is under control after ten treatments. No recurrence during follow-up.

Notes: The plum-blossom needle is effective for treating migraine. Migraine due to cold should be treated twice a day. Mild and superficial stimulation is used on the patient's head, if there is ascendant hyperactivity of liver yang. Heavy tapping should be done on points lateral to C1, and on positive reaction points on the superclavicular fossa, to cause bleeding. Bloodletting therapy is given every other day, depending on the patient's condition, for beneficial effect.

External application therapy

Patient Liu is a 31-year-old woman.

The patient has suffered from recurrent headache on the left side for eight years. The pain becomes severe as a result of tiredness and emotional disturbance. The pricking pain is severe. It is accompanied by amaurosis, nausea, and vomiting. Diagnosis given by the specialist hospital is migraine. The patient used to take ergotamine and carbamazepine to relieve pain. The medication has lately failed to relieve pain. The patient also has stomach problems after taking the medication. The tongue is pale, with thin, white coating. The pulse is wiry and tight.

Diagnosis: Migraine.

Acupoints: Nose, head, on the affected side.

Manipulation: Pound herbal medicine Chuanxiong (*Rhizoma Chuanxiong*), Baizhi (*Radix angelicae dahuricae*), Qianghuo (*Rhizoma et radix notopterygii*) and Xixin (*radix et rhizoma asari*) to a fine powder. Place the powder on a piece of absorbent cotton, and roll it up to the diameter of the nostril. Place the medicated roll into the left nostril, and keep it there for 20–40 minutes.

Pound herbal medicine Chuanxiong (*Rhizoma Chuanxiong*), Baizhi (*Radix angelicae dahuricae*), Qianghuo (*Rhizoma et radix notopterygii*), Fangfeng (*Radix saposhni-koviae*), Jiangcan (*Bombyx batryticatus*), Juhua (*Flos chrysanthemi*), Gaoben (*Rhizoma ligustici*), Cansha (*Faeces bombycis*), Manjingzi (*Fructus viticis*) and Bingpian (*Borneolum syntheticum*) – which is packed in a single bag – to power and put it into a container. Close the container with a piece of kraft paper. Heat the container over strong fire for ten minutes. After boiling the herbs, put Bingpian (*Borneolum syntheticum*) into the hot water, and then steam the left side of the head with the container for ten minutes. The treatment is given three times with one bag of herbal medicine, every other day, and ten times forms a course of treatment. No recurrence has been reported.

Effect: The pain is relieved on the same day.

Notes:

- The herbal medicine is given via acupoints for instant effect, combining the effect of the medicine and the acupoints. The nostril-medicine therapy and steaming therapy are combined for quick effect on the affected region.

- The above-mentioned therapy can be effective when used alone.

- Herbal poultice can also be used in the treatment. Pound Shengnanxing (raw *Rhizoma arisaematis*), Shengwutou (raw *Radix aconiti*), Baizhi (*Radix angelicae dahuricae*), and Xixin (*Radix et rhizoma asari*) to a fine powder and mix them with onion juice into a paste. Put the paste on EX-HN-5 Taiyang on the affected side. The external application is changed every day.

Collateral pricking and bloodletting therapy

Patient Li is a 41-year-old man.

The patient has suffered from headache on the left side for 20 years. The left-side headache is due to excessive use of the brain in his youth. The pain is recurrent and accompanied by tinnitus, and vexing heat in the chest, palms, and soles. No organic change is revealed by examination. The patient has been on all kinds of pain-relieving drugs, for a long time. The pain has recently become severe, and now causes blurred vision.

Blood vessels are visible on EX-HN-5 Taiyang. The color of the lips is dark. The tongue is enlarged with stagnated blood. The pulse is thready and unsmooth.

Diagnosis: Migraine due to blood stasis.

Acupoints: EX-HN-5 Taiyang on effected side.

Manipulation: Disinfect the skin in the normal way. Prick the acupoint with a three-edged needle and collect 5ml blood.

Effect: Headache is relieved after treatment. The patient took pain-relieving medication only once in the week following acupuncture treatment. (He used to take medication every day.) Bloodletting therapy is used on EX-HN-5 Taiyang on the left side and LU-5 Chize, in the second treatment. Headache and tinnitus are relieved in the following week. The patient still feels distension on the head. Bloodletting therapy is used on EX-HN-5 Taiyang on the left side, on the apex of the ear, and on veins posterior to the ear, in the third treatment. No recurrence is reported during follow-up.

Notes: Many factors cause migraine, including hypertension, stress, poor blood supply to the head, poor sleep, and muscle dysfunction of the head and the neck.

Bloodletting with a three-edged needle can be used on certain acupoints of the body. A small amount of stagnated blood or tissue fluid is expelled from the local area to improve circulation and treat disease. Bloodletting on EX-HN-5 Taiyang, LU-5 Chize, BL-40 Weizhong, the apex of the ear, veins posterior to the ear, and Jiangyagou brings good results.

EX-HN-5 Taiyang is located in the depression one finger-width posterior to the meeting point of the eyebrow and the outer canthus. Search for collaterals in that area, and prick them with the three-edged needle to a depth of 2–3 fen. Ask the patient to lower his head when the blood comes out. Put a cup over the point to collect the blood.

Remove the cup and clean the point when the bleeding stops.

Three points should be noted when pricking EX-HN-5 Taiyang:

- *First*, the muscle layer on this point is thin. Therefore, prick the needle to a depth of 2–3 fen and avoid inserting a needle so deeply on this point that it touches the bone.

- *Second*, tie a towel round the neck to make the vein stand out and then prick it.

- *Third*, feel the beating temple artery and avoid puncturing the artery.

Ask the patient to stand holding on to a chair to support the body during bloodletting on BL-40 Weizhong. Search for the area with obvious collaterals. If the collaterals are not clear, then prick the point 1–2 fen above or on the left or right. Disinfect the acupoint. Hold the knee steady with the left hand, and prick with the three-edged needle in the right hand, to a depth of 2–3 fen. Withdraw the needle and cover the point with a cup. Remove the cup when bleeding stops.

Two points require attention:

- *First*, avoid pricking veins inferior to BL-40 Weizhong, even prominent veins, since many patients have difficulty walking after pricking on that point.

- *Second*, hold the knee still with the left hand to prevent the patient moving it (when the needle would prick normal tissue).

The cephalic vein passes through LU-5 Chize. The collaterals are on the lateral side of the cubital crease. Prick with the three-edged needle to a depth of 2–3 fen. Withdraw the needle and cover the point with a cup to collect blood.

Warm silver needle

Patient Xu is a 32-year-old woman. Her first consultation is on 19 June 2007.

The patient has suffered from recurrent headache on the right side of the head for three years. The headache started in spring 2004, due to overwork and irregular lifestyle. The recurrent distension pain on the right side of the head becomes severe as a result of stress or tiredness. The pain abates after rest. The patient has tried all kinds of modern medicine and Chinese medicine, but without effect. The patient presents with distension and throbbing pain in the right side of the head. The pain attacks 6–8 times per week. It is accompanied with dryness of both eyes, or sometimes with tears. The patient has poor sleep; she sleeps about four hours every night. No abnormality is found in neurological examinations.

Diagnosis: Migraine.

Manipulation: Insert small silver needles on the origin and the insertion of the trapezius muscle and pyramidalis muscle. The insertion is 3cm inferior to the lower border of the occipital tuberosity and the superior nuchal lines on both sides, and touches the periosteum. About six needles are used in this part of the treatment. Three more needles are inserted posterior to the mastoid, on the insertion of the splenius capitis muscle and the semispinalis capitis muscle. Needles are inserted 0.5cm lateral to the spinous process, from C2 to C5. Wrap moxa around the end of the needle handle and perform warming needle moxibustion until the end of the treatment.

Effect: The patient's headache is obviously relieved after acupuncture treatment. The treatment is given every other week. Headache is relieved after three treatments. No headache occurs during two-year follow-up.

Notes: Silver needle therapy (developed by Professor Xuan Zheren) is effective in treating soft tissue disorders. 0.5 percent lidocaine is injected into the local point to form a 5mm high protuberance from the skin. Then insert the silver needle perpendicularly into the affected area, as far as the periosteum, to cause a strong needling sensation of soreness, distension, and numbness. Wrap moxa around the end of the needle handle and perform warming needle moxibustion for 20 minutes. Withdraw the needle when it is cool. The punctured area should not come in contact with water for three days, to prevent infection.

Combined acupuncture treatment

Patient Geng is a 34-year-old woman. Her first consultation is on 16 July 2002.

The patient has suffered from severe distension and pain on the right side of the head for eight years. She takes sedative and pain-relieving medicine orally to reduce the pain. The patient lost her job half a year ago. She cannot get to sleep at night, and the headache becomes severe. It is also accompanied by irregular menstruation. The pain affects her work and daily life severely. All examination results are normal.

The patient presents with severe pain on the right side of the head. The pain radiates to EX-HN-5 Taiyang. It is accompanied by poor sleep, irregular menstruation, restlessness, and dry mouth. Tender points are found on the right temple, forehead, and the apex of the head. The tongue is red with thin, white coating. The pulse is thready and uneven.

Diagnosis: Migraine.

Treatment: EX-HN-5 Taiyang (right), GB-20 Fengchi (right), penetrating needling from SJ-23 Sizhukong (right) to GB-8 Shuaigu, RN-4 Guanyuan, KI-12 Dahe, SJ-5 Waiguan, GB-41 Zulinqi. Mild stimulation is used on local acupoints, and strong manipulation on distal acupoints. Needles are retained for 30 minutes. Put a TDP lamp (mineral lamp that uses far infrared light emissions to increase microcirculation) over the low abdomen during the treatment.

- Prick and squeeze for 10 drops of blood on both the ear apex and EX-HN-5 Taiyang on the right side.

- Tap the plum-blossom needle with moderate to strong power on Hua Tuo Jiaji points, especially on points with nodules of positive reaction. Tap the region for 15 minutes.

- Apply seeds to ear acupoints, such as Temple, Occipital, Subcortex, Shenmen, and Sympathetic Nerve.

Effect: Most of the pain is relieved after one treatment. Administration of sedative and pain-relieving medicine is stopped. All the symptoms are relieved after ten treatments. The treatment is repeated ten times to maintain the effect. There is no recurrence during one-year follow-up.

Acupuncture combined with herbal medicine

Patient Wu is a 25-year-old woman. Her first consultation is in the year 2000.

The patient has suffered from migraine on the right side for about 10 years. Acupuncture treatment relieves the pain during an attack. The severe headache is recurrent, due to emotional disturbances. The pain continues for the entire day and is accompanied by symptoms of nausea, vomiting, dizziness, distension, restlessness, short temper, and poor sleep. The patient sleeps for only four hours every night, or not at all. The patient also has abdominal distension, poor appetite, dry mouth, yellow urine, and dry stools. The tongue is red, with pale yellow coating. The pulse is deep and thready. The patient has had irregular menstruation for four years, and once had amenorrhea for three months; she took Chinese medicine and luteosterone to cure this.

Diagnosis: Migraine (irregular menstration).

Acupoints: EX-HN-5 Taiyang on the affected side; SP-6 Sanyinjiao, RN-12 Zhongwan, LR-14 Qimen, and GB-20 Fengchi on both sides.

Manipulation: Manipulate the needle with neutral reinforcement and reduction. Needles are retained for 30 minutes. Prick EX-HN-5 Taiyang on the right side for blood. The treatment is given once a day.

This is a long-term case. Strong medicine should not be used when eliminating pathogens. The patient should treat the headache gradually by taking some pills made from Chinese herbs. The prescription is as follows.

> Pao Fuzi (prepared *Radix aconiti lateralis praeparata*) 30g, Danggui (*Radix Aagelicae sinensis*) 30g, Chuanxiong (*Rhizoma Chuanxiong*) 20g, Gouqizi (*Fructus lycii*) 20g, Tianma (*Rhizoma gastrodiae*) 20g, Gaoben (*Rhizoma ligustici*) 20g, Jiangbanxia (*Rhizoma pinelliae praeparatum*) 20g, Chaobaizhu (prepared *Rhizoma atractylodis macrocephalae*) 20g, Fuling (*Poria*) 20g, Chaozaoren (prepared *Semen ziziphi spinosae*) 20g, Zhi Dawugong (prepared large *Scolopendra*) 10 pieces, Zhi Quanxie (prepared *Scorpio*) 20g.

Pound the above-mentioned herbs into a fine powder. Mix the powder with honey and make it into pills the size of the little fingernail. Take the medicine in 3g doses, three times a day.

Effect: Headache is relieved after acupuncture; however, there will be mild recurrence following treatment. Therefore, herbal medicine is used to gradually treat the disease. After two months' medication, the headache is cured; the menstruation is also regular.

Notes:

- Acupuncture and herbal medicine have their own advantages. Acupuncture is good at regulating meridians and treating exterior problems. Herbal medicine is effective in adjusting interior Zang-Fu organ disorders. Acupuncture is used to relieve pain and treat the symptoms, and herbal medicine to treat the cause of headache. In this case, acupuncture is used first to relieve pain. Then herbal medicine is given to maintain the effect.

- The pill contains insects which are effective at dispelling pathogens from the meridians. Herbs with the effect of harmonizing the middle and extinguishing wind are also combined in the prescription. This treatment is effective in both the short and the long term.

- This is the experienced prescription of Dr. Zhang Cigong. It is effective in treating severe headache, and good at treating migraine related to menstrual disorders. The prescription can be used without modification.

Tuina manipulation

Patient Zhao is a 48-year-old woman. Her first consultation is on 15 September 2001.

She complained of amphicrania (headache affecting both sides of the head) and dizziness for five years, soreness in the neck, numbness in the scalp, insomnia, reluctance to open eyes; there was no nausea or vomiting, no deafness or tinnitus. On palpation, tenderness was found around the transverse process of C2; there was also stiffness in the muscles around the neck, and tenderness behind the mastoid. CT of the cerebral cranium: normal. X-ray of the cervical vertebrae: overstraightening showed cervical curve, narrowing of the intervertebral space, hyperostosis of the vertebral edge, abnormal shape of intervertebral foramen, and misalignment of the odontoid process. Several kinds of Chinese and Western medicine had been used without satisfactory therapeutic effect. Pathological changes inside the brain, inflammation, diseases of the five sensory organs, hypertension, and hyperlipemia were excluded.

Diagnosis: Migraine (cervical).

Treatment: The patient was in a sitting position, with the practitioner standing on the affected side. The manipulations were applied in three steps.

- Applied one-finger-pushing back and forth from EX-HN-3 Yintang to ST-8 Touwei, EX-HN-5 Taiyang, along the hairline on forehead, for 3–4 times; then applied pressing and kneading on EX-HN-3 Yintang, BL-1 Jingming, EX-HN-4 Yuyao, DU-20 Baihui, EX-HN-5 Taiyang, etc.

- Applied grasping along the five channels from the vertex to BL-10 Tianzhu and GB-20 Fengchi, then grasped along the Bladder Meridian to both sides of DU-14 Dazhui, back and forth, 4–5 times, and wiped the forehead 3–5 times. After that, finger-kneading was done on the muscles around the neck and shoulder.

- Finally, with the patient lying on her back, the practitioner performed rotational manipulation of cervical vertebra on fixed point. The practitioner stood at the bedside, with one hand pressing one side of patient's face and the other hand holding the occipital area, and asked the patient to relax. Hook-pushing and pulling were applied on the spinal process of C2 with the index finger; the transverse process of C2 on the same side was pushed with the thumb, and the patient's head was forced through the maximum rotation to one side with the assistance of the other hand. Then both hands gave strength simultaneously, and a plucking sound was heard. After the manipulation, some kneading and pressing were applied for a while.

Note: If the spinal process of C2 is crooked towards the left, rotate the head to right and push the transverse process on the left side. If it is crooked towards the right, push the transverse process on the right side.

Effect: After the first treatment, the headache was relieved; the eyes were bright; the feeling of relaxation was like offloading a huge stone from head. After three sessions of treatment, it was cured and never relapsed.

Notes: Migraine of cervical origin indicates migraine induced by strain and stiff muscles around neck, degeneration of cervical vertebrae, intervertebral joint replacement, distortion of the intervertebral foramen, intervertebral disk hernia, destabilization of cervical vertebrae, and displacement of joints, especially damage to the atlanto-axial joint, which can induce pain, spasm, and pressure on muscles around neck, or stimulate the major and minor occipital nerve, major auricular nerve, and nearby blood and sympathetic nerves. Manipulations are applied to relax sinews and activate collaterals, and to relieve muscle spasm around neck, with stimulation on GB-20 Fengchi, EX-HN-5 Taiyang, BL-10 Tianzhu, DU-20 Baihui to disperse wind and activate collaterals, clear the mind, and relieve pain.

One-finger-pushing

Patient Wu is a 43-year-old woman with 11 years of migraine on the right side, with weekly attacks of over ten hours' duration, stabbing pain, nausea, and dizziness; frequent analgesia is ineffective; distending epigastric pain continued for several months and was relieved after stopping administration of drugs; she had thirst and a bitter taste in the mouth, bad odor, poor appetite, constipation, and yellow urine. Examination showed lack of vitality, no varices on the head, tenderness on the occipital bone, EX-HN-5 Taiyang, ST-8 Touwei, and the supraorbital ridge; red tongue with yellow coating; wiry and slippery pulse.

Diagnosis: Migraine.

Treatment: The patient was in a sitting position, and slightly closed her eyes; the practitioner stood by her side. The therapy mainly used one-finger-pushing and rolling. There were four steps:

- Held the occipital region with one hand, and applied one-finger-pushing with the other hand along the Gallbladder Channel and the five meridians on the head and face region, i.e. on the forehead, from EX-HN-3 Yintang to DU-23 Shangxing; on the forehead, from EX-HN-3 Yintang to EX-HN-5 Taiyang; on Qiaogong (cleidomastoid); on the area around the orbits; on the temple, from ST-8 Touwei to EX-HN-5 Taiyang, to ST-6 Jiache.

- Applied grasping on the vertex, with the middle finger pointing towards the Governor Channel, and the other four fingers along the Gallbladder Meridian and Bladder Meridian. The manipulation was repeated several times, from the forehead to the occipital area.

- The practitioner applied rolling on the neck and nape region with one hand, meanwhile using the other hand to assist the head in passive exercises; also applied pressing on GB-20 Fengchi, DU-16 Fengfu, BL-10 Tianzhu; grasping on the muscles on the nape, GB-21 Jianjing, SJ-5 Waiguan, LI-4 Hegu; point-pressing on GB-34 Yanglingquan and LR-3 Taichong.

- Applied kneading with the outer flank of the thumb on the surface projection of the sympathetic trunk in the anterior region of the neck and carotid artery. The whole therapy was no more than 40 minutes, once a day; 20 times forms a course of treatment.

Effect: Pain was relieved after five sessions of treatment with slight manipulations. After two courses of treatment, the condition was cured. No relapse was reported in the follow-up.

Notes:

- According to legend, one-finger-pushing was first introduced by Bodhidharma, and became popular in Song Shan and Luo Yang in Henan province. The manipulation was passed on to Ding Fengshan in the late Qing dynasty, and then refined by his son, Ding Jifeng.

- The key points of the manipulation are: put the finger tip, the flank, and the tip of radialis of the thumb on the channel points or regions, relax the shoulder and elbow joints, and exert a constant force on the channels, points, and regions by means of continuous swinging of the wrist and flexion and extension motions of the thumb joints.

- Ding Jifeng then created rolling after years of dedication. The key points of the manipulation are: place the region of the palm near the small finger on the treatment area, flex the metacarpo-phalangeal joints a little, and make that part of the palm do continuous movement back and forth by means of maximum flexion and extension of the wrist joint. The focus of contact should be on the treating area, and the force should be even and penetrating.

- Tuina therapy can release muscular tension, restore functionality of vasomotion, improve circulation, increase blood supply to the head, and adjust functionality of nerves and blood vessels, so that migraine is relieved.

Chapter *6*

Summary of Treatments

Section I Acupuncture for Treating Migraine

Migraine is a common condition for which there are various kinds of acupuncture treatment. General treatment, medication, subperiosteal blockage of the temporal bone, and stellate (inferior cervical) ganglion blockage, and other methods besides, are used to treat migraine. Healthy lifestyle, stable mood, and regular exercise are necessary, while foods that can trigger migraine (such as coffee, oranges, and chocolate) are forbidden during general treatment. Medication used to treat migraine includes analgenics (such as aspirin, naproxen, ibuprofen, and indomethacin), vasoconstrictors (like ergotamine) and enteramine agonists (like sumatriptan). Subperiosteal blockage of the temporal bone is commonly used: 5ml indomethacin is injected from EX-HN-5 Taiyang into the subperiosteal of the temporal bone, at an angle of 45 degrees. This can produce marked improvement in one or two treatments, and cure in four treatments. Another effective therapy is stellate ganglion blockage using lidocaine. In addition, bloodletting, auricular acupuncture, moxibustion, plum-blossom needles, scalp acupuncture, and abdominal acupuncture are also used to treat migraine. Acupuncture, moxibustion and massage are widely accepted because of the easy manipulation, rapid effect, low cost and absence of side-effects.

There is a large body of clinical research on acupuncture treatment for migraine. In one report from Australia, pain decreased by more than 33 percent and medication decreased by 40 percent, following acupuncture. The overall success rate for migraine treated by acupuncture is 93.8 percent, compared to

62.5 percent treated by Western medicine, according to a report from Harbin, China.

Experience in point selection

Treatment of migraine by acupuncture is discussed in *Huangdi Neijing*: "Cold migraine is treated by the Hand-Shaoyang-Meridian and Hand-Yangming-Meridian, and by the Foot-Shaoyang-Meridian and Foot-Yangming-Meridian," said *Lingshu Jing* (*Miraculous Pivot*). After thousands of years' development, rich experience of best practice has been accumulated, such as point selection by *syndrome differentiation*, point selection by *meridian differentiation*, point selection by *distant and near differentiation*, and point selection by *experience*.

POINT SELECTION BY SYNDROME DIFFERENTIATION

Syndrome differentiation is important. According to this principle, treatment is formulated based on one of the following syndromes: exopathy, internal injury, cold, heat, deficiency, and excess. This is the key point in treatment. Point selection by syndrome differentiation aims to dispel the basic cause of migraine, which can achieve a stable result.

The doctor must grasp the essential characteristics, distinguish the syndrome, and determine therapy according to clinical presentation and the course of pathogenesis. This means that different therapies are used on cold, heat, and damp syndromes – the main principle when treating exogenous headache is to reduce unhealthy qi, such as cold, heat, and dampness. Internal injury headache may require:

- treating liver yang hyperactivity with liver-calming and liver-yang-suppressing therapy

- treating renal and blood deficiency with reinforcing methods

- treating turbid phlegm with phlegm-dispelling and dampness-eliminating therapy

- treating blood stasis with stasis-dispelling therapy.

Headache that lasts for a long time and resists cure is called head wind (Toufeng), and for this, activating collaterals and wind-dispelling therapy should be used.

Dispelling humidity and cold-dispersing therapy is used to treat wind-damp headache, which is caused by head wind (Toufeng) along with humidity.

- **Wind-cold headache:** GB-20 Fengchi, DU-16 Fengfu, BL-12 Fengmen, SI-3 Houxi, BL-65 Shugu; apply uniform reinforcing–reducing manipulation, slight sweat on head is a good sign.

- **Wind-heat headache:** DU-14 Dazhui, GB-20 Fengchi, LI-4 Hegu, LU-7 Lieque; reducing manipulation.

- **Humidity headache:** SP-6 Sanyinjiao, ST-40 Fenglong, SJ-10 Sidu; uniform reinforcing-reducing manipulation.

- **Humidity-heat headache:** SP-6 Sanyinjiao, SJ-10 Sidu, ST-40 Fenglong, LU-7 Lieque; add Xing-points or Shu-points to clear excess heat humidity, uniform reinforcing–reducing manipulation.

- **Cold-humidity headache:** SP-6 Sanyinjiao, ST-40 Fenglong, LR-3 Taichong, PC-6 Neiguan; reinforcing manipulation, moxibustion after acupuncture.

- **Turbid-phlegm headache:** LI-6 Pianli, LU-7 Lieque, ST-40 Fenglong, SP-4 Gongsun, PC-6 Neiguan; uniform reinforcing–reducing manipulation.

- **Qi-deficiency headache:** ST-36 Zusanli, RN-6 Qihai, RN-12 Zhongwan, DU-20 Baihui; reinforcing manipulation, moxibustion after acupuncture.

- **Xue-deficiency headache:** LR-3 Taichong, KI-3 Taixi, GB-39 Juegu, LU-7 Lieque; uniform reinforcing–reducing manipulation.

- **Liver-fire headache:** GB-44 Zuqiaoyin, LR-2 Xingjian, GB-20 Fengchi, BL-63 Jinmen; reducing manipulation.

- **Blood-stasis headache:** RN-17 Danzhong, BL-17 Geshu, GB-41 Zulinqi; uniform reinforcing–reducing manipulation, with increased needle retention and qi-promotion.

- **Toufeng headache:** BL-63 Jinmen, GB-20 Fengchi, LR-3 Taichong, KI-3 Taixi, GB-41 Zulinqi, DU-16 Fengfu; uniform reinforcing–reducing manipulation.

POINT SELECTION BY MERIDIAN DIFFERENTIATION

The main meridians running over the head include three yang meridians and the Foot-Jueyin-Meridian. Pathogenic factors attack via the meridians. The basis for migraine treatment is *syndrome* differentiation. There are many other locations for migraine apart from the sides of the head. *Meridian* differentiation is used to guide point selection and description, whatever the pathogenic factors and syndromes are. It is useful to apply meridian differentiation and Zang-Fu differentiation techniques, as Zang-Fu differentiation has important directional significance.

Note: Zang-Fu differentiation is different from meridian differentiation in acupuncture and moxibustion therapy. Manipulation is strict on this particular point.

- **Shaoyang headache:** GB-41 Zulinqi, SJ-5 Waiguan, auxiliary with SJ-23 Sizhukong through EX-HN-5 Taiyang.

- **Yangming headache:** ST-44 Neiting, LI-4 Hegu, auxiliary with ST-14 Yangbai, EX-HN-3 Yintang.

- **Taiyang headache:** BL-60 Kunlun, SI-3 Houxi, auxiliary with GB-20 Fengchi, BL-10 Tianzhu.

- **Jueyin headache:** LR-3 Taichong, PC-6 Neiguan, auxiliary with DU-20 Baihui.

SJ-5 Waiguan and GB-41 Zulinqi belong to the Shaoyang Meridian. LI-4 Hegu and ST-44 Neiting belong to the Yangming Meridian. SI-3 Houxi and BL-60 Kunlun belong to the Taiyang Meridian. PC-6 Neiguan and LR-3 Taichong belong to the Jueyin Meridian. The points listed above belong to the meridians of same name.

Yang meridians connect in the face and head, while yin meridians connect in the chest and abdomen, and the meridian qi channels cross one another. This means that selecting points on the meridians with the same name is useful as they have corresponding functions.

Professor Jin Bohua thinks that reverse qi disturbing the orifices, and failing to nourish the brain, is the main pathogenesis of migraine. Treatment by meridian differentiation based on pain location is a common and effective clinical practice.

Treat *excess syndrome* with effusing Shaoyang therapy; and treat *deficiency syndrome* with nourishing yin and soothing liver yang therapy of Shaoyang headache.

Treat *excess syndrome* with GB-41 Zulinqi and LR-3 Taichong, using the reducing method, and KI-3 Taixi, using uniform reinforcing–reducing manipulation. Treat *deficiency syndrome* with KI-3 Taixi, using reinforcing therapy, and GB-41 Zulinqi, using reducing therapy; then auxiliary techniques with GB-8 Shuaigu, GB-20 Fengchi, DU-20 Baihui, SJ-20 Jiaosun, ST-8 Touwei, EX-HN-5 Taiyang, BL-2 Cuanzhu, LU-7 Lieque.

Treat *excess syndrome* with reconciliation, clear and descending therapy of Yangming headache. Choose SP-1 Yinbai, SP-4 Gongsun, RN-12 Zhongwan using reducing method; then auxiliary techniques with SP-6 Sanyinjiao, ST-36 Zusanli, and PC-6 Neiguan according to syndromes such as loose stool, deficiency qi and sloth, feebleness. Treat *deficiency syndrome* with reinforcing spleen and kidney therapy. Choose left SP-6 Sanyinjiao, right KI-3 Taixi, ST-36 Zusanli, and RN-12 Zhongwan; then apply auxiliary techniques with EX-HN-3 Yintang, EX-HN-5 Taiyang, ST-8 Touwei, DU-22 Xinhui, and LI-4 Hegu. Add RN-6 Qihai for women, and RN-4 Guanyuan for men. Needling points on the feet and legs have beneficial effect in migraine.

Treat *excess syndrome of Taiyang headache* with BL-60 Kunlun, GB-39 Juegu, and SP-6 Sanyinjiao, using reducing therapy; KI-3 Taixi, using reinforcing therapy; DU-16 Fengfu, DU-15 Yamen, using pricking therapy; then apply auxiliary techniques with GB-20 Fengchi, BL-10 Tianzhu, GB-11 Touqiaoyin, and EX-HN-1 Sishencong. Treat *deficiency syndrome* with KI-3 Taixi, using reinforcing method; and BL-60 Kunlun, using reducing method; then auxiliary with SI-6 Yanglao, SJ-3 Zhongzhu, GB-20 Fengchi, GB-11 Touqiaoyin.

Soothing the liver and lowering adverse qi, dredging collaterals, and relieving pain are used to treat Jueyin headache. LR-3 Taichong and LR-2 Xingjian; then auxiliary with GB-39 Juegu and EX-HN-1 Sishencong, are usually chosen.

Syndrome differentiation based on meridian differentiation is effective under direction of using reducing therapy for sthenic syndromes and reinforcing therapy for asthenic syndromes.

POINT SELECTION BY DISTANT AND NEAR DIFFERENTIATION

There are also criteria for selecting points that lie a) near the affected region, or b) at a distance from it.

For obvious and immediate pain relief, select EX-HN-5 Taiyang through GB-8 Shuaigu, DU-20 Baihui through GB-5 Xuanlu, and ST-8 Touwei through GB-7 Qubin – based on point selection near the affected region. Another prescription consists of EX-HN-5 Taiyang, GB-20 Fengchi, DU-20 Baihui, SJ-23 Sizhukong through GB-8 Shuaigu, and ST-8 Touwei. Local points can be chosen if there is obvious pain. GB-20 Fengchi is the preferred point, DU-16 Fengfu and Ashi points are secondary.

Selecting distant points is better than selecting points near the affected region. SJ-2 Yemen and GB-39 Xuanzhong are used to treat pain in the temporal area; add KI-16 Huangshu for pain in the prefrontal cortex; add BL-63 Jinmen for occipital headache referred to the temples.

SJ-6 Zhigou and GB-41 Zulinqi are used to treat Shaoyang headache: select SJ-6 Zhigou, and perform manipulation after inserting the needle, until qi arrives. Add GB-41 Zulinqi if the pain persists.

According to our experience, points on the limbs can be selected to treat headache without fixed location, and this agrees with the view of Professor Jin Guanyuan: he thought that stimulating the central reflection area on the limbs (area in the limbs that is connected with the brain), instead of points on head, can treat headaches in cases where the patient cannot pinpoint the location of it.

Distant point selection can also be used to treat headache with obvious disease location.

Both distant and local point selection are used to treat stubborn migraine and complicated headache:

- GB-20 Fengchi, EX-HN-5 Taiyang, ST-8 Touwei, GB-38 Yangfu, and GB-43 Xiaxi are used to treat migraine attributed to the Shaoyang Meridian.

- DU-23 Shangxing, EX-HN-3 Yintang, BL-2 Cuanzhu, and LI-4 Hegu are used to treat frontal pain attributed to the Yangming Meridian.

- GB-20 Fengchi, BL-10 Tianzhu, SI-3 Houxi, and BL-60 Kunlun are used to treat occipital headache attributed to the Taiyang Bladder Channel of the Foot.

- DU-20 Baihui, BL-7 Tongtian, GB-20 Fengchi, and LR-3 Taichong are used to treat parietal pain attributed to the Jueyin Liver Channel of the Foot.

THE IMPORTANCE OF BRANCH AND ROOT

It is important to distinguish between branch and root in treating migraine with acupuncture.

For *acute and heavy head pain*, headache controlling therapy should be used, which means controlling branch syndromes in an emergency condition, where an acute and heavy headache is beginning. GB-39 Juegu on the affected side is usually used to treat migraine; add Ashi points and LI-4 Hegu if there is supraorbital ridge pain; add LU-7 Lieque if there is parietal pain; add SI-3 Houxi and DU-16 Fengfu if there is occipital headache. Auricular acupuncture, ophthalmic acupuncture, and scalp acupuncture are used if those don't work.

As to *chronic headache*, syndrome differentiation is important. Root syndromes should be considered in chronic conditions. LR-3 Taichong and LR-2 Xingjian are used to soothe excessive liver yang; ST-40 Fenglong and SP-9 Yinlingquan are used to eliminate dampness and resolve phlegm.

Because of the relationship between pathogenic factors and headache attack, branch and root should be treated together. Multiple needles and acupoints and long-term therapy are used to treat acute attacks of chronic headache.

POINT SELECTION BY EXPERIENCE

There is much unique clinical experience of treating migraine with acupuncture other than by Zang-Fu differentiation and meridian differentiation. This is called point selection by experience.

According to syndrome, lesion site, and meridian, Wang Le Ting (creator of the Golden Needle method of acupuncture) gives acupuncture based on octo-acupuncture of headache, an experienced prescription of Wang, consisting of DU-20 Baihui, EX-HN-5 Taiyang, DU-16 Fengfu, GB-20 Fengchi, and LI-4 Hegu.

SJ-23 Sizhukong through GB-8 Shuaigu is used by Professor He Puren to treat migraine simply by pricking EX-HN-9 Neiyingxiang. Add BL-67 Zhiyin if there is occipital headache. Add ST-44 Neiting if there is prefrontal headache.

Professor Xu Benren is expert in using GB-20 Fengchi. Insert the needle towards the contralateral eyeball, and perform twirling and twisting, lifting and thrusting manipulations with strong stimulation until there is a needling sensation of numbness and expansion. Press the muscle below GB-20 Fengchi with left thumb, meanwhile continue manipulating the needle with the right hand until needling sensation radiates to EX-HN-5 Taiyang or the calvaria.

GB-20 Fengchi, a point of Shaoyang Gallbladder Channel of the Foot, has the function of dispelling wind to relieve exogenous syndrome, relieving the head and improving eyesight.

Professor Yang Zhaogang inserts an elongated needle, directed towards the contralateral eyeball, to a depth of 1.5–2 cun, and manipulates it until the needling sensation reaches the calvaria and forehead – with good results.

Professor Wei Jia is good at treating migraine using BL-67 Zhiyin.

EX-HN-5 Taiyang can be used to treat acute attacks of migraine, according to Liu Guanjun: one needle is inserted perpendiculary into the point; the other is inserted into the point directed towards the zygomatic arch, so with oblique needling. Headache may cease as soon as qi is obtained.

Professor He Shuhuai usually selects a Hua Tuo paravertebral point, such as T5, T7, T9, T11, or T14, to regulate the function of the relevant Zang-Fu organ, and GB-20 Fengchi to stimulate meridian qi on the head as well.

Experience in needle manipulation

Acupuncture is the main therapy for treating migraine; pricking therapy, auricular acupuncture therapy, moxibustion, and electro-acupuncture therapy are secondary. "Compared to acupoint, obstacle of acupuncture exist in manipulation," said Li Shouxian, an acupuncturist during the Qing dynasty. Manipulation is an essential component for obtaining qi (and clinical success). Only proper manipulation can create the right needling sensation, which is both a precondition and a guarantee of clinical success.

Strong fingers are required for an acupuncturist to manipulate needles successfully. Relax the mind, the arm, and the fingers. Exert force the moment you insert and begin to manipulate the needle. Soothing but strong fingers are important for producing good needling sensation. After inserting the needle, it is best to manipulate it so as to create needling sensation and for it to be conducted from one area to the other, which is fundamental for good results.

Controlling qi and regulating the meridians is the key to acupuncture, according to Professor Ma Ruilin – i.e. it is the managing of needling sensation and induction that regulates the flow of meridian qi fluency, and restores correct functioning of the human body. Twirling and twisting, lifting and thrusting, and thrilling the needle, massaging meridians, pinching and pressing techniques, are used singly or in combination on the right meridian points to stimulate needling sensation, which is important in inducing meridian qi and promoting clinical effect.

Reducing therapy with longer needle retention and intermittent manipulation or electro-acupuncture, is usually used to treat headache. It is combined with moxibustion for asthenia and cold syndrome. Intradermal needles on effective points can be used to maintain stimulation after the headache has been alleviated.

Needling technique for migraine varies between proximal points and distal points. Slight stimulation should be used on local points, and can cause slight soreness and distension. SJ-23 Sizhukong through GB-8 Shuaigu are commonly used points. Be deft when inserting needles through the scalp, and careful when inserting needles along it. Stop inserting if there is any resistance or pain; withdraw the needles from one to two points, and then reinsert them. Do not insert a needle by forcing it, to avoid suffering.

EX-HN-5 Taiyang is another commonly used point. Insert the needle into EX-HN-5 Taiyang and towards GB-8 Shuaigu, at an angle of 15 degrees and to a depth of 2 to 2.5 cun. Twirl and twist for one minute after the patient senses, for example, soreness and distension in the temples, and the headache will stop immediately.

Strong stimulation should be used for distal points so that needling sensation is conducted to the lesion site.

Electro-acupuncture can be used to help control headache.

Many experts emphasize the use of GB-20 Fengchi in treating migraine. Insert the needle towards the contralateral eyeball for about 1.2 cun, twirling and twisting it consistently until there is a sensation of soreness and distension in the occiput, or radiating to the forehead. Manipulate the needle every ten minutes for 30–40 minutes.

There is another technique in which the needle is inserted into the ligamentum flavum until the patient has an electrical sensation. The pain will stop the moment the needle is withdrawn.

Other special experience

Integration of meridian differentiation and Zang-Fu differentiation is fundamental in treatment for migraine. Different therapies are used on cold, heat, and damp syndromes, following the main principle of reducing unhealthy qi when treating exogenous headache. For headache due to internal causes:

- treat liver yang hyperactivity so as to calm the liver and suppress liver yang

- treat kidney and blood deficiency with reinforcing methods

- treat turbid phlegm by dispelling phlegm and eliminating dampness

- treat blood stasis by dispelling stasis.

Persistent headache that resists cure is called Toufeng. Activate collaterals and dispel wind to treat this kind of headache.

Dispel humidity and disperse cold to treat wind-damp headache.

Treatment based on syndrome differentiation auxiliary with GB-20 Fengchi is effective.

In addition, there are different kinds of headache, such as Yangming headache, Shaoyang headache, Taiyang headache, and Jueyin headache, related to different pain sites and characteristics such as frontal, parietal, and occipital pain. Different points and manipulations should be selected, based on meridians and organs.

"Needling lower to treat upper" has special effects in migraine. A major pathogenic factor in headache, is qi failing to circulate or flow upwards and downwards. "Needling lower to treat upper" can regulate qi activity, increase lucidity and decrease turbidity.

Reducing therapy is used to treat sthenia, with the function of clearing pathogenic factors through the feet and refreshing the head and eyes.

Reinforcing therapy is used to treat asthenia, with the function of regulating yin and yang, and raising qi to nourish the head and eyes. KI-3 Taixi is selected to treat headache because the kidneys control bone, generate marrow, and connect with the brain.

Migraine caused by high blood pressure in the head can be treated with blood-letting therapy on EX-HN-5 Taiyang or the superficial veins in the temples.

Migraine related to menstruation can be treated by needling reaction points near SP-6 Sanyinjiao, SP-9 Yinlingquan, LR-8 Ququan, BL-27 Xiaochangshu and BL-31 Shangliao, BL-32 Ciliao, BL-33 Zhongliao, and BL-34 Xialiao.

In treatment for tension migraine, reaction points arround the trapezius muscles and acupoints such as BL-19 Tianzhu, GB-20 Fengchi, DU-14 Dazhui, SI-15 Jianzhongshu, BL-13 Feishu, GB-21 Jianjing, and SI-13 Quyuan decrease at the same time as the headache is alleviated.

Application of experience

Acupuncture has a positive effect on migraine. Headache may stop the moment needles are inserted. Because of variation in patients' sensitivity, integration of several acupuncture techniques, or rotational use of acupuncture techniques, may be more effective. So acupuncture, warming acupuncture, bloodletting therapy, auricular acupuncture, and prescription of Chinese herbs, etc., can be used in combination. Doctors should master the maximum possible number of acupuncture techniques, so as to obtain the best results in the shortest time.

Acupuncture has rapid effect in treating migraine, while prescription of Chinese herbs is radial treatment. Chronic migraine should be treated with acupuncture combined with prescription. Liquid acupuncture therapy can be selected if this doesn't work.

Tianma (Chinese herb injection) is injected into acupoints such as GB-20 Fengchi, EX-HN-5 Taiyang, Ashi points, LI-4 Hegu, BL-2 Cuanzhu, EX-HN-3 Yintang, Anmian, and SJ-17 Yifeng. Injecting 1 percent procaine hydrochloride into Ashi points is effective for both acute and chronic migraine. The dosage is 0.5ml per point, once a day.

Section II Tuina for Treating Migraine

Tuina therapy for treating migraine consists mainly of the manipulations of pushing, grasping, point-pressing, wiping, rubbing, and tapping to soothe the sinews, harmonize qi and blood, open orifices, and refresh vitality, so as to restore brain vasomotion and improve circulation, by which means migraine can be cured. The acupoints formula for Tuina is similar to that for acupuncture, varying according to Zang-Fu differentiation and meridian differentiation. The method for each manipulation on specific acupoints also has strict requirements. Mastering each method and applying them fluently will augment benefit from treatment.

Selecting acupoints for Tuina

The acupoints selected for Tuina in the treatment of migraine are similar to those for acupuncture. The methods used for selecting acupoints are discussed below.

BASIC METHOD FOR ACUPOINT SELECTION

Migraine pain is mainly located in the head, and especially on one side. The key to therapy is to treat according to disease location, and to apply the right kind of therapy. The basic method is to give therapy in light of patients' symptoms to treat the key area of disease location.

Methods:

- Open Tianmen (push from EX-HN-3 Yintang to the anterior hairline).
- Push Kangong (push from EX-HN-3 Yintang along both eyebrows).
- Press EX-HN-5 Taiyang and the mastoid process, grasp GB-20 Fengchi, press DU-20 Baihui, LI-4 Hegu, and the Ashi points.

DIFFERENTIATION ACCORDING TO ETIOLOGY AND DISEASE

Apart from the basic method, differentiation should be made according to the etiology and disease mechanism of different patients. There are four main types of differentiation manipulation.

Ascendant hyperactivity of liver yang

Headache and distension on one side, flushed complexion with red eyes, irritated and agitated state, red tongue with yellow coating, and wiry pulse. Apply pressing on acupoints SJ-20 Jiaosun, GB-8 Shuaigu, ST-8 Touwei, and grasping on GB-21 Jianjing.

Ascendant turbid phlegm

Headache and distension on one side of the head, nausea, reduced appetite, sticky, white phlegm, white and greasy tongue coating, slippery pulse. Apply rubbing on acupoints RN-12 Zhongwan, BL-20 Pishu, and apply pressing on ST-36 Zusanli and ST-40 Fenglong.

Yin deficiency of liver and kidneys

Headache on one side, dizziness, lumbar weakness and soreness, vexing heat in the chest, palms, and soles, blurred vision, red tongue with sparse coating, thready and wiry pulse. Apply rubbing on acupoints RN-6 Qihai, RN-4 Guanyuan, and BL-23 Shenshu.

Obstruction of brain collaterals

Relapse of headache on one side, stabbing pain in fixed location for long periods, purple tongue with thin, white coating, thready and uneven pulse. Apply pressing, kneading, and wiping on EX-HN-5 Taiyang, BL-2 Cuanzhu, and other points located in the forehead and head along the Gallbladder Meridian.

ALONG-MERIDIAN DIFFERENTIATION

Apart from the head, patients with migraine may also feel pain in other locations, and so meridian differentiation is made in Tuina therapy, to instantly relieve pain. The following acupoints along meridians are commonly applied: EX-IIN-5 Taiyang, GB-8 Shuaigu, DU-20 Baihui, GB-5 Xuanlu, ST-8 Touwei, GB-7 Qubin, SJ-23 Sizhukong, GB-9 Tianchong, GB-20 Fengchi.

- *For Shaoyang headache,* distant acupoints of SJ-5 Waiguan, SJ-6 Zhigou, GB-41 Zulinqi, GB-39 Juegu, and local acupoints of GB-20 Fengchi, GB-8 Shuaigu, SJ-20 Jiaosun, EX-IIN-5 Taiyang, and SJ-23 Sizhukong are commonly used.

- *For Yangming headache,* distant acupoints of ST-44 Neiting, LI-4 Hegu, and local acupoints of EX-HN-4 Yuyao, GB-14 Yangbai, ST-8 Touwei, and EX-HN-3 Yintang are used.

- *For Taiyang headache,* distant acupoints of BL-60 Kunlun, SI-3 Houxi, and local acupoints of GB-20 Fengchi and BL-10 Tianzhu are used.

- *For Jueyin headache,* distant acupoints of LR-3 Taichong, PC-6 Neiguan, and local acupoints of DU-20 Baihui and EX-HN-1 Sishencong are used.

Strict rules apply to Tuina manipulations. When using distant acupoints, the kneading and pressing should conduct sensation from the wrists and ankles to the arms and legs.

Some experience of Tuina manipulation

Differentiation should be introduced when applying Tuina manipulation. Depending on the different size and depth of the disease location, different manipulations are applied to cover the pain area and stimulate various layers of tissue. Also, methods vary according to location; for example, grasping and plucking are used on tendons; pressing, point-pressing, and fingernail pressing are applied to acupoints and pressure points; manipulations such as shaking and pulling to take joints through a range of passive movements, are used to treat joint problems.

The commonly used manipulations for treating migraine are pushing, grasping, point-pressing, wiping, rubbing, and tapping. A basic procedure is that of opening Tianmen (pushing from EX-HN-3 Yintang to the hairline), then pushing Kangong (wiping and pushing from EX-HN-3 Yintang to the supraorbital ridge), transporting and transforming qi in EX-HN-5 Taiyang, kneading the protruding bone behind the ear, grasping GB-20 Fengchi, and point-pressing DU-20 Baihui, LI-4 Hegu, and the Ashi points.

The correct method of Tuina manipulation is vital for therapeutic benefit, and the general requirements are proficiency, agility, soft, even, persistent, and forceful manual technique, and conveying power from the surface to the internal environment. During Tuina the movement of manipulation should be coherent, power should be consistent, and the period of treatment proportionate, so that the area being treated responds well and patients find the treatment acceptable. Inappropriate manipulation would both reduce therapeutic benefit and upset patients' psychologically, resulting in a poor prognosis.

The main manipulations for treating migraine, applied on the face and head, are as follows.

- **Grasping five meridians:** Grasp with thumb and four fingers from the vertex to the occiput; next, apply five finger-grasping on GB-20 Fengchi, and then grasp along either side of the cervical vertebrae down as far as C7. Repeat the process 3–5 times.

- **Pushing Qiaogong:** Push Qiaogong with the thumb. Push one side of the acupoint up and down 20–30 times, then push the other side.

- **Face and head region:** Steady the patient's head with one hand and use the thenar of the other hand to push and wipe from the middle of the forehead to the occipital region for two minutes; then point-press BL-2 Cuanzhu, GB-14 Yangbai, SJ-23 Sizhukong, EX-HN-5 Taiyang, ST-8 Touwei, SJ-20 Jiaosun, GB-8 Shuaigu, GB-12 Wangu, GB-20 Fengchi, and DU-20 Baihui. Each acupoint should be pressed for around one minute. Repeat the process 1–2 times.

- **Dispersing:** Push with top of the thumb along the Gallbladder Meridian, from the forehead to the back of the head. Repeat the process on each side, at least 20 times. Strength of manipulation should be adjusted according to the type of headache: for deficiency syndrome, apply soft strength and slight stimulation; excess syndrome should be treated with more forceful manipulation and stronger stimulation, within a range that is acceptable to patients. By way of example, we will take SJ-5 Waiguan and GB-41 Zulinqi to illustrate manipulation on distant acupoints.

  ○ **Pressing and kneading SJ-5 Waiguan:** With the patient in supine position, and the practitioner standing beside the bed, use the thumb to press and knead SJ-5 Waiguan on both sides, either simultaneously or alternately. Continue pressing for 1–2 minutes, in a slightly upwards direction, achieving the corresponding sensation in the arm.

  ○ **Pressing and kneading GB-41 Zulinqi:** With the patient in supine position and the practitioner standing beside the bed, use thumb pressing on GB-41 Zulinqi, with the tip of the thumb pointing towards the ankle, and the other four fingers holding the foot. Press in the direction of the heel for 1–2 minutes, until achieving the corresponding sensation in the ankle.

- Just as in acupuncture, many experts emphasize the importance of manipulation on GB-20 Fengchi. Commonly used manipulations are kneading, pressing and scrubbing.

  ○ With the patient in supine position, and the practitioner sitting beside the patient's head, use the hands or thumbs to push, wipe, press, and knead the uncomfortable areas around the orbit and forehead. Then use the middle fingers of both hands to knead GB-20 Fengchi, the fingers pointing towards the forehead, and the thenar holding the temporal side. Strength should be gradually increased to achieve the corresponding sensation in the forehead and temple; maintain strength for 2–3 minutes, then apply kneading to release strength; finally, use the thumb to push from GB-20 Fengchi to the shoulder, and relax the shoulder with grasping.

Other unique experience

Different practitioners have different experience of Tuina manipulation for treating migraine; some stress meridian differentiation, others Zang-Fu differentiation, but all attach importance to local therapy. Tuina manipulation is given on the basis of local therapy, according to the theory of meridians and collaterals, and differentiated according to Yangming headache, Shaoyang headache, Taiyang headache, and Jueyin headache. Essentially, migraine is internal diseases manifesting via the meridians and collaterals onto the surface of the body. Hence, the correct manipulations are based on proper differentiation of Zang-Fu and meridians.

According to Traditional Chinese Medicine, stagnation of qi and blood causes pain, and when stagnation is elminated, pain will be relieved. So applying pressing, kneading, flicking, and plucking on spasm "hotspots" in the temples will soothe meridians and activate blood, move qi and relieve pain. The process is as follows: the practitioner uses the index fingers or middle fingers of both hands to search for spasm around the temples on either side, and then applies pressing, kneading, flicking, and plucking on the spasm spot for 3–5 minutes to relieve it.

Clinical research shows that dislocation of the spine relates to migraine, to some extent. When treating some migraine patients who also have cervical spondylopathy or misaligned spinous processes of thoracic vertebrae, treatment should first be given to realign the spine, so that benign stimulation will then be conducted to the corresponding ganglia. Restoring normal functions of the spine will help to balance the state of qi and blood.

Proper application

Tuina manipulation is effective for treating migraine. Some treatment might achieve instant pain relief following pressure, but in most cases a combination of manipulations and systematic treatment is required. It is evident that etiology, pathology, and patient's constitution and sensitivity to therapy differ among individuals, so if results are not satisfactory with one manipulation, others need to be used, and combination with acupuncture might be better. Different manipulations are selected according to duration of treatment and disease location. Only by mastering a range of treatments using acupuncture and Tuina can practitioners achieve the best results in the shortest time.

We believe that Tuina combined with ear point therapy produces convincing results.

Section III Precautions and Prognosis

Precautions

LIFESTYLE HABITS

If migraine patients correct unhealthy lifestyle habits, this will contribute much to relieve the duration and intensity of migraine.

Patients should adopt a healthy routine, with a good balance between work and relaxation, avoiding frequent late nights, so as to guarantee good rest. Lack of sleep, drowsiness, and irregular sleep are major factors in migraine, so guaranteeing good sleep is an important avoidance strategy. Also, if encountering pressure or emotional disturbance in daily life, patients should unwind emotionally by chatting with friends, listening to music, or participating in sport or outdoor activities, so as to relieve pressure and dispel unhealthy emotions.

Patients need to avoid taking contraceptive drugs, vasodilators, hormonal, surrenal, and ergotamine medications, in order to prevent drug-induced migraine.

On the subject of diet, it is better if patients avoid food that contains tryptophan, tyrosine, and glutamic acid, and alcoholic drinks such as spirits and red wine, and drinks that contain caffeine, such as coffee, cola and tea. Proper eating habits and regular mealtimes are important, to avoid hunger or over-consumption of food. Limiting the use of monosodium glutamate also helps to prevent migraine.

Patients need to avoid negative environmental factors such as cold wind, overexposure to sun, harsh light, dry heat, dampness, peculiar smell, excessive noise, polluted air, and radiation.

Avoiding unhealthy reading habits and quitting tobacco will help to prevent migraine.

Treatment given before or after menstruation, for female patients whose disease is related to menstruation, is beneficial.

SELF-TREATMENT

For most migraine patients, movements such as head exercises and climbing stairs will aggravate headache, so activities involving these should be avoided.

Pressing on the carotid artery, or eyeball, or pulling the hair, bedrest and napping will reduce pain.

Dipping the hands in warm water reduces pain effectively for most migraine patients. At the beginning of the onset stage, dip both hands in warm water. (The temperature should be comfortable.) Keep adding warm water to keep the temperature up and dip for around 20 minutes.

There are some other folk remedies that bring benefit in treating migraine, such as cupping on EX-HN-5 Taiyang until the local skin turns dark purple; scraping the neck and back with a coin until red spots appear; pinching the forehead or EX-HN-5 Taiyang to produce purple spots.

Migraine prognosis

Acupuncture is beneficial in treating migraine, especially for those patients with migraine of short duration and strong intensity. Exogenous headache usually has immediate onset, and relapse after cure is rare. Migraine due to internal factors requires careful syndrome differentiation; otherwise, although symptoms may be relieved after acupuncture, some patients will experience relapse. If acupuncture is combined with oral administration of Chinese medicine, the benefit will be increased.

However, acupuncture has little effect on migraine that is complicated by a brain tumor or cerebral hemorrhage, so imaging is needed before treatment with acupuncture, to exclude particular conditions and guarantee optimal therapy for different patients.

All in all, proper application of acupuncture and Tuina, with clear differentiation of disease, achieves good therapeutic results.

References

1. *Huangdi's Internal Classic Plain Questions*. Beijing: People's Medical Publishing House, 1978.

2. *Miraculous Pivot*. Beijing: People's Medical Publishing House, 1979.

3. Yang Jizhou. *The Great Compendium of Acupuncture and Moxibustion*. Beijing: People's Medical Publishing House, 2006.

4. Qiu Maoliang. *Chinese Therapeutics of Acupuncture and Moxibustion*. Nanjing: Phoenix Science Press, 1988.

5. Shao Shuijin. *WeiJia's Experiences on Acupuncture and Moxibustion*. Shanghai: Shanghai University of Traditional Chinese Medicine Press, 1999.

6. Xiao Shuchun. *Essence of Mordern Acupuncture Literature*. Beijing: Chinese Traditional Chinese Medicine Ancient Books Publishing House, 1988.

7. Beijing Traditional Medicine Training Center of the World Federation of Acupuncture and Moxibustion Societies. *Experiences of Famous Old Experts on Acupuncture and Moxibustion*. restricted material.

8. Chen Youbang. *Modern Essence of Clinical Acupuncture and Moxibustion in China*. Beijing: China Press of Traditional Chinese Medicine, 1986.

9. Zhou Meisheng. *Moxibustion Thread*. Qingdao: Qingdao Publishing House, 2006.

10. Huang Lichun. *Ear points Therapy*. Beijing: Scientific & Technological Literature Publishing House, 2005.

11. Plum-blossom Needle Section, Acupuncture and Moxibustion Dept., Guang'anmen Hospital, China Academy of Traditional Chinese Medicine. *Plum-blossom Needle Therapy*. Beijing: People's Medical Publishing House, 1973.

12. Zhong Meiquan. *Chinese plum-blossom needle*. Beijing: People's Medical Publishing House, 1998.

13. Wu Zhenxi. *Internal Diseases Treated with External Therapy in Chinese Medicine*. Beijing: People's Medical Publishing House, 2007.

14. Chen Keji. *Essence of Formulas for External Therapy in Qing Dynasty*. Beijing: People's Medical Publishing House, 1996.

15. Wang Xiuzhen. *Therapy of Pricking Blood*. Hefei: Anhui Scientific & Technological Publishing House, 1985.

16. Zheng Pei. *Mirror of Pricking Blood*. Hefei: Anhui Scientific & Technological Publishing House, 1999.

17. Wang Zheng. *The Complete Compendium of Therapies of Pricking Blood*. Hefei: Anhui Scientific & Technological Publishing House, 2005.

18. Du Huaitang. *The Complete Compendium of Proven Formulas of Modern Famous Doctors in China*. Shijiazhuang: Hebei Scientific & Technological Publishing House, 1990.

19. Ding Jifeng. *The Great Compendium of Tuina*. Zhengzhou: Henan Scientific & Technological Publishing House, 1997.

20. Song Wenge. *Practical Clinical Pain*. Zhengzhou: Henan Scientific & Technological Publishing House, 1997.

21. Sun Shentian. *New Practical Clinical Verses of Acupuncure*. Beijing: People's Medical Publishing House, 2007.

22. Jin Guanyuan. *Clinical Acupuncture Reflexology*. Beijing: Beijing Scientific & Technological Publishing House, 2004.

23. Jin Bohua. *Essence of Jin's Clinical Acupunture*. Beijing: People's Medical Publishing House, 2005.

24. Wang Qicai. *Acupuncture and Moxibustion Therapy*. Beijing: Chinese Traditional Chinese Medicine Ancient Books Publishing House, 2003.

25. Zhang Xinshu. *Practical Wrist-ankle Needle Tharapy*. Beijing: People's Medical Publishing House, 2002.

26. Bo Zhiyun. *Abdomen Needle Tharapy*. Beijing: China Science and Technology Press, 1999.

27. Yin Yuanping. *The Complete Works of Chinese Special Method of Acupunture*. Shenyang: Liaoning Scientific & Technological Publishing House, 2000.

28. He Puren. *Clinical Application of Acupuncture-Moxibustion Three Removing Obstruction Methods*. Beijing: Scientific & Technological Literature Publishing House, 1999.

29. Wang Lvsheng. *Doctor of Clinical Chinese Medicine-Wang Leting*. Beijing: China Press of Traditional Chinese Medicine, 2005.

30. Zhong Lan. *Tuina to Treat Pain*. Beijing: Scientific & Technological Literature Publishing House, 2001.